Samaneh Sheibani
Somayeh Sheibani

Scientific Study of Patients

Samaneh Sheibani
Somayeh Sheibani

Scientific Study of Patients

with Uterine and Cervical Lesions

Noor Publishing

Imprint
Any brand names and product names mentioned in this book are subject to trademark, brand or patent protection and are trademarks or registered trademarks of their respective holders. The use of brand names, product names, common names, trade names, product descriptions etc. even without a particular marking in this work is in no way to be construed to mean that such names may be regarded as unrestricted in respect of trademark and brand protection legislation and could thus be used by anyone.

Cover image: www.ingimage.com

Publisher:
Noor Publishing
is a trademark of
Dodo Books Indian Ocean Ltd., member of the OmniScriptum S.R.L Publishing group
str. A.Russo 15, of. 61, Chisinau-2068, Republic of Moldova Europe
Printed at: see last page
ISBN: 978-620-3-86036-8

Scientific Study of Patients with Uterine and Cervical Lesions

By

Dr. Samaneh Sheibani

Gynecologist, Member of the Elite National Foundation, Infertility and IVF fellowship, Top Rank and Assistant Professor of Shahid Beheshti University of Medical Sciences, Tehran, Iran

Dr. Somayeh Sheibani

Gynecologist and has a Specialized Board, Ahwaz University of Medical Sciences, Iran

This Book is dedicated to

My Family's

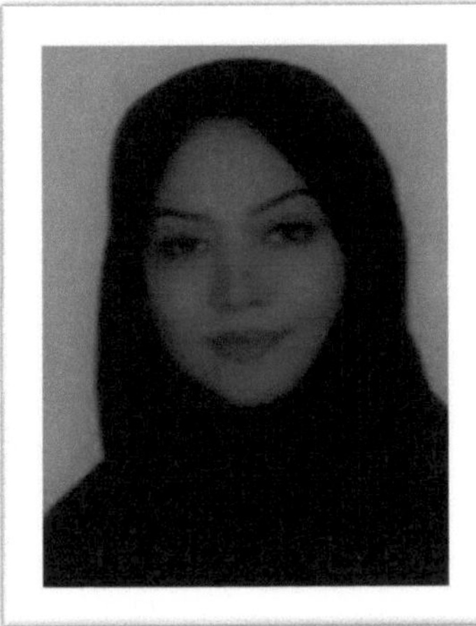

Dr. Samaneh Sheibani

Gynecologist, Member of the Elite National Foundation, Infertility and IVF fellowship, Top Rank and Assistant Professor of Shahid Beheshti University of Medical Sciences, Tehran, Iran

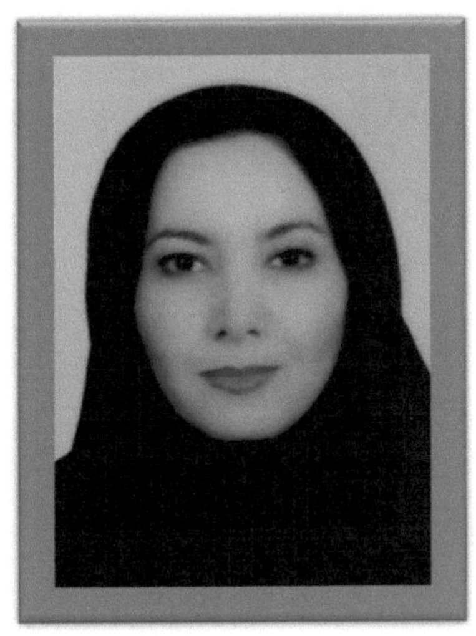

Dr. Somayeh Sheibani

Gynecologist and has a Specialized Board, Ahwaz University of Medical Sciences, Iran

Content

Chapter I

Introduction

Chronic Service

Chronic cervicitis is extremely common and tends to affect the junction of the squamous-cylindrical epithelium in the cervix and is sometimes accompanied by hyperemia, edema, fibrosis, and metaplastic changes. PID is a complication of pregnancy. Common organisms are responsible for HSV and chlamydia, but syphilis, amoebiasis, and actinomycosis are also rare. In many cases, no specific organism is identified, but cellular pathological changes appear to be more pronounced in a group with clinical symptoms (in the form of mucoid-purulent discharge) and a specific organism separated from the culture of the discharge.

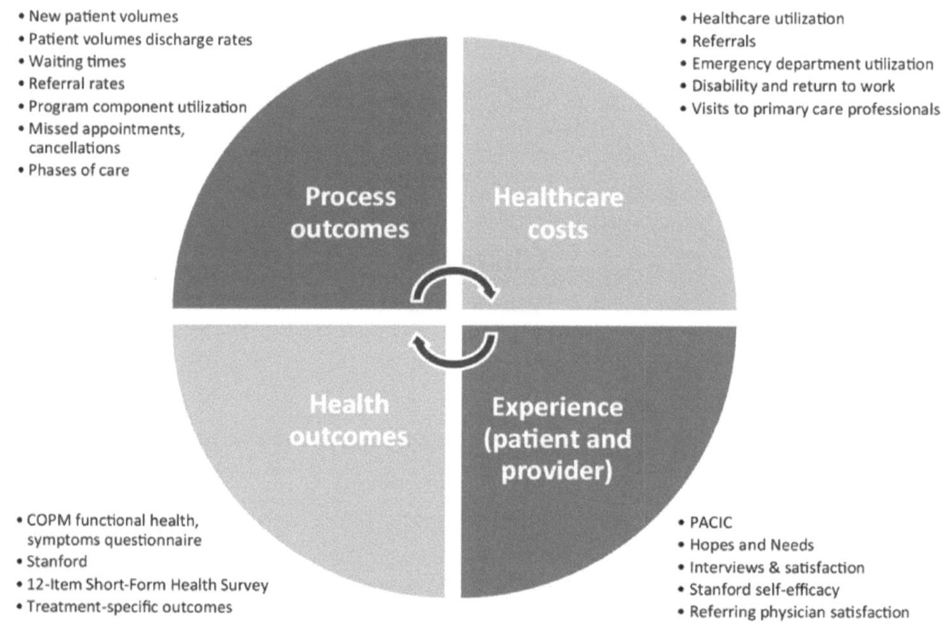

Figure 1. Integrated Chronic Care Service (ICCS)

Cervical polyps

Endocervical polyps are benign inflammatory tumor lesions that are seen in 2- 5% of women in puberty. These polyps are often small and are derived from chronic polypoid services. These lesions require differentiation from more dangerous lesions due to abnormal vaginal bleeding (often in the form of spotting). The superficial epithelium of these lesions is often metaplasia, but the incidence of intraepithelial neoplasia of the cervix (CIN) is not higher than in other normal areas of the cervix, and in most cases, simple curettage or removal of polyps by surgery can eliminate the complications.

Cervical metaplasias

Different types of metaplasia occur in the cervix, the characteristics of each of which are related to the type of tissue involved. Squamous metaplasia is the most common type of cervical metaplasia that occurs at the junction of two squamous and cylindrical epithelium in the cervix. Other types of cervical Mtaplazyhay include transitional cell metaplasia, tubular metaplasia, intestinal metaplasia and intestinal metaplasia Lvlhay- The first is Sngfrshyy epithelium endocervical glandular epithelium exocervix and the rest of squamous metaplasia seen Myshvd.astlah stratified squamous epithelium when used as a substitute for glandular epithelium Has been. This finding is so common in the cervix that it is practically considered a normal finding. Almost all women of childbearing age have some degree of squamous metaplasia. In most cases, the lesion involves the superficial part of the epithelium so that the endocervical glands are covered by squamous cells. In advanced degrees, the epithelium of the affected area is indistinguishable from the exocervical epithelium.

Cervical Cancers

Cervical squamous cell neoplasms

Fifty years ago, cervical carcinomas were the leading cause of death for women with cancer in most countries, but today the mortality rate for women with cervical cancer has dropped to two-thirds, followed by lung, breast, colon, pancreas, and ovarian cancers. Lymph nodes and blood are in eighth place. This success owes much to the invention of Pap smear and other new diagnostic methods and their widespread use in recent decades. The cervix is almost always derived from the junction of the squamous epithelium and the cylinders of the cervix (Transformation). This lesion is slow-growing and remains in non-invasive stages for many years.

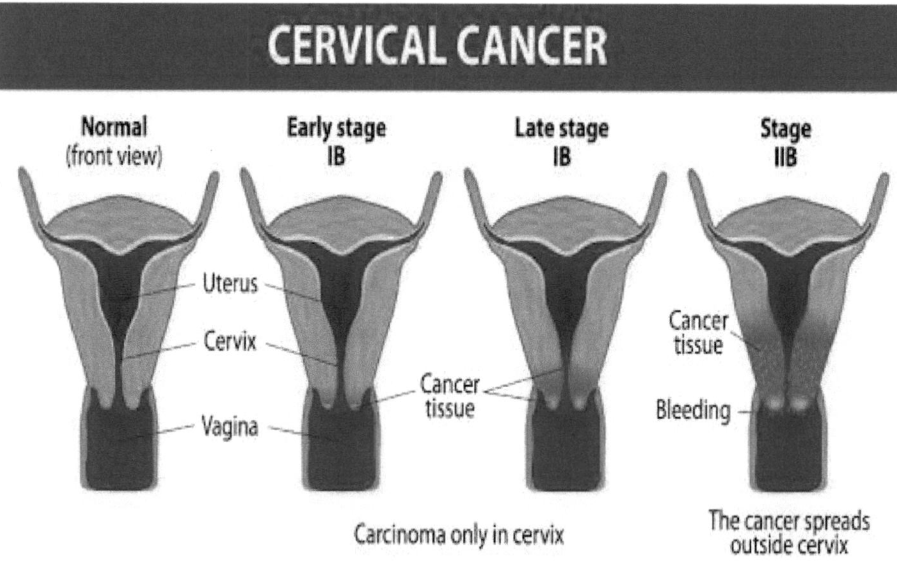

Figure 2. Cervical cancer

It has been shown that the incidence of this lesion is significantly related to a person's sexual activity, so that it is almost never seen among nuns, and the main risk factors for developing this lesion are:

1. The young age of the person at the beginning of sexual activity
2. Having multiple sexual partners
3. Having a male sexual partner who has been in a relationship with several sexual partners.

In this regard, human papillomavirus (HPV) is the most important factor in the oncogenicity of cervical lesions. HPV is a DNA virus with 60 different types and today is responsible for a range of cervical diseases from benign lesions such as Condyluma acuminatum. Malignancy is known as squamous cell sinus function. The virus is sexually transmitted and prefers metaplastic tissues. Among the 60 different types of the virus, infections of types 44, 42, 11, 6 are more common, but it seems that infection with types 31, 16, 18 is more dangerous and causes the lesions become high grade. In addition to the clear association between HPV and CIN and squamous cell carcinomas, there is now evidence that the virus is associated with other cervical neoplasms such as adenocarcinomas and adenosquamous carcinomas.

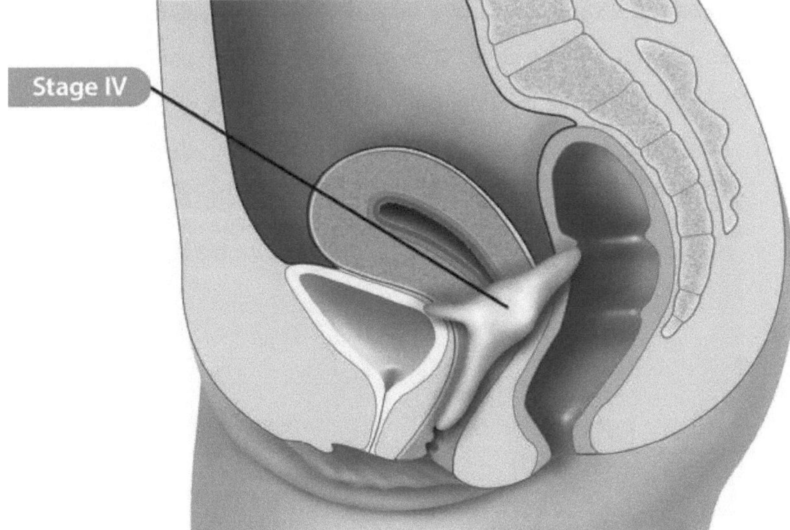

Figure 3. A Guide to Cervical Cancer, Symptoms, Causes, Prevention, and Treatments

Although the role of the HPV virus in the development of cervical cancers has been proven, evidence shows that of the many women with a history of infection with the virus (75% of all women), only about 10% have intraepithelial neoplasms (CIN) and a small percentage (3/3). 1% develop invasive carcinoma. In addition, in a percentage of CIN cases, not only does the lesion not progress to invasive carcinoma, but the lesion also stops and regresses. It is for cervical neoplasms. There is still no definite agreement on the effects of OCP and other hormones such as diethyl acetylbestrol on the course of these lesions. When a pathologist diagnoses CIN in a cervical biopsy specimen, it is the responsibility of the obstetrician to determine the presence or absence of invasive carcinoma, which of course is of great therapeutic importance for high-grade lesions.

Treatment

In the past, hysterectomy was used as the only initial treatment for CIN, but since research has shown that 99.7% of cervical dysplasias (including in situ carcinoma) are confined to a depth of 3.8 mm above the surface of the cervical epithelium, surgical methods are now more conservative. It is considered a disease, but in any case, hysterectomy is still one of the treatment methods in recurrent or high-grade cases of these lesions, especially in people who do not want to maintain their fertility.

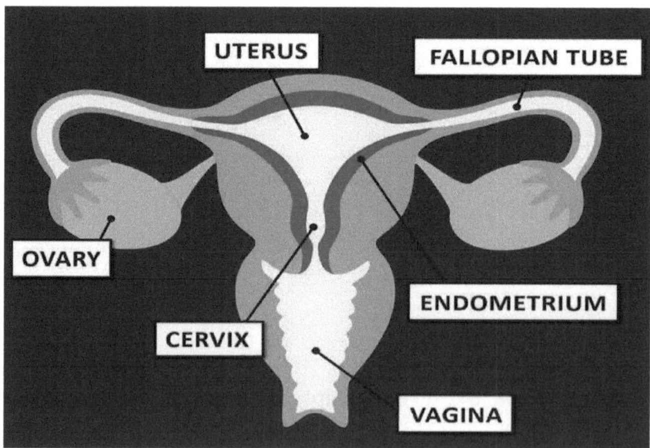

Figure 4. Does Cervical Cancer Run in Families?

Cervical squamous cell carcinoma (SCC)

Despite the reduction in SCC mortality, this lesion is still the most common female genital malignancy in most parts of the world. SCC occurs at any age from20 to old age, but the most common age of onset in invasive lesions is 40 to 45 years. In high-grade precancerous lesions, it is 30 years old. Today, due to the widespread use of 1-smear method and perhaps the decrease in the age of first sexual contact in young people, the average age of these lesions is decreasing. Cervical cancer is slow and usually remains without a clinical symptom for a long time, so in many cases the lesion It is found during screening tests or accidentally in cases of hysterectomy performed due to another lesion. In the advanced and invasive stages of the disease, abnormal vascular pattern and other structural changes in the affected cervix cause spotting, abnormal bleeding, dyspareunia, dysuria, and leukorrhea. They are classified in a separate group called micro invasive squamous cell carcinoma. These lesions, which often correspond to stage IA in the FIGO system, are more similar to high-grade CIN (in situ carcinoma) and differ in clinical course and treatment from other invasive cervical carcinomas. These lesions almost always originate at the site of an early CIN and are often located at the anterior edge of the cervix. Recent studies show that this group of cervical carcinomas leads to lymphatic metastases in only 1% of cases and the main criterion for differentiating these lesions and estimating the probability of lymph node metastasis is tumor volume.

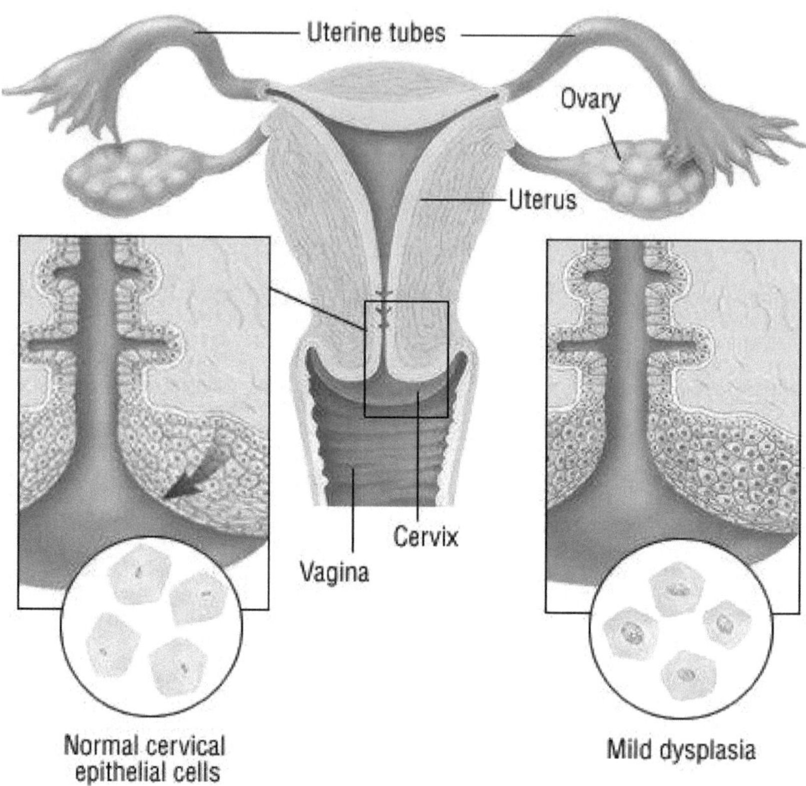

Figure 5. Cervical Cancer Guide: Causes, Symptoms and Treatment Options

Staging

Stage o: On-site carcinoma (carcinoma insitu)

Stage I: Limited lesion of the cervix

Stage II: The lesion extends beyond the cervix but does not reach the pelvic wall or affects the vaginal tumor but does not affect the lower third.

Stage III: The tumor has spread to the pelvic wall and there is no healthy distance between the tumor and the pelvic wall on rectal examination.

Stage IIV: The lesion extends beyond the pelvis or involves the bladder and rectal mucosa.

How it spreads and metastasizes

Cervical carcinomas mainly spread directly to adjacent organs (uterus, vagina, lower urinary tract, and eutrosacral ligaments), but lymph node metastasis is also common, but blood metastases are rarely reported to distant organs (often bony).

Treatment and Prognosis

Treatment of invasive cervical lesions, depending on the extent of the lesion and the patient's general condition, may include surgery, radiation therapy, or a combination of the two. Invasive lesions are often treated with hysterectomy, and in advanced lesions radiotherapy is performed. In cases where a latent invasive carcinoma is discovered accidentally after a hysterectomy, radical reoperation is usually required, followed by surgical resection of the lesions.

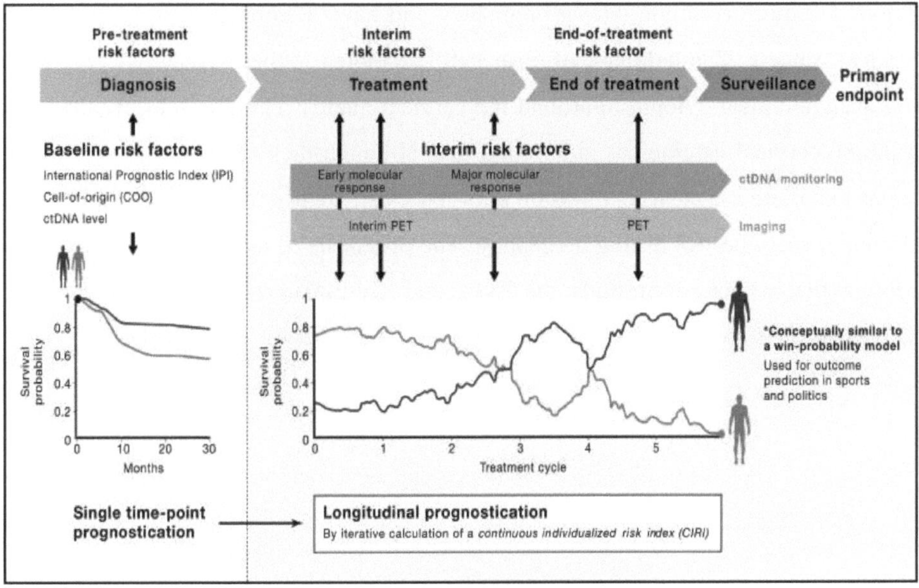

Figure 6. Hey CIRI, What's My Prognosis?

If no remedial effects are observed within 1 to 3 months, concomitant chemotherapy is also considered. The prognosis and survival rate of patients mainly depends on the stage of the lesion at the time of discovery and with existing treatments, the 5-year survival rate for stage I is between 80. Up to 90%, for stage II 75%, for stage III about 35% and for stage IV about 10 to 15%. Other adenosquamous carcinomas, clear cell carcinoma Undifferentiated carcinomas make up a total of 25% of all cervical cancer lesions. they give. Cervical adenocarcinomas account for 5-15% of all cervical cancer lesions. Adenocarcinomas of the cervix make up 5-15% of all cervical carcinomas. This rate is higher in Jewish women, while the prevalence of SCC in this group is lower than the normal population. Some sources equate the origin of SCC, adenocarcinoma, and adenosquamous lesions of the cervix. (Ackerman's p.1371) But in other sources, endocervical cells have been introduced as the source of adenocarcinomas. (Robbin's pathologic basis diswase p.1053). Adenocarcinomas have many similarities to SCC, but appear to be more associated with HPV18 and occur at older ages than SCC. Adenosquamus carcinoma has both squamous and glandular components. These lesions are more common during pregnancy and have a worse prognosis than other cervical cancers. The hallmark of clear cell carcinoma is the presence of cells with abundant and clear cytoplasm around the cervical glands. These lesions are the most common cervical carcinomas at a young age, although they can occur at any age. It seems that there is a clear relationship between the incidence of this lesion and the use of diethyl acetylbestrol during pregnancy. The prognosis of these lesions is relatively good, so that in a long-term study, the 5-year and 10-year survival rates of patients with this lesion were 55% and 40%, respectively.

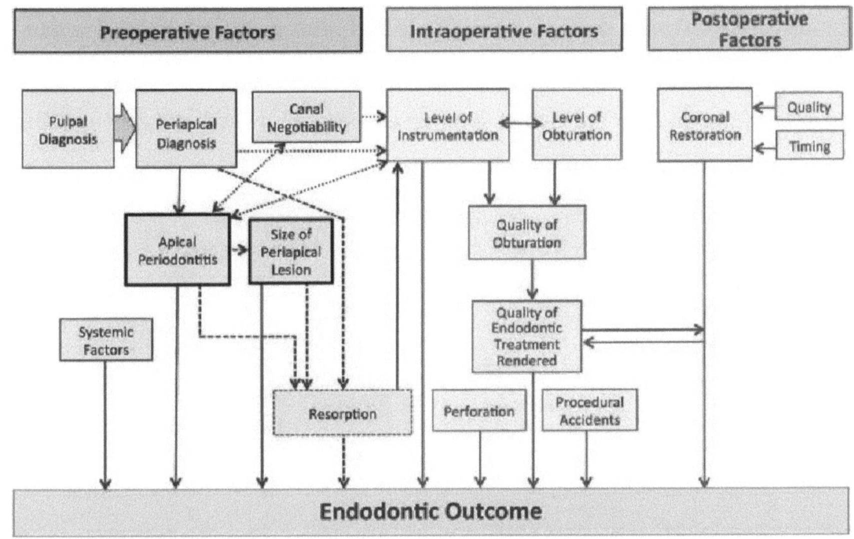

Figure 7. Endodontic Prognosis Clinical Guide for Optimal Treatment Outcome

Pathological lesions of the uterus

Endometritis

Unlike cervicitis, which is a common and insignificant finding, due to the protective role of the cervix and the anatomical condition of the uterus associated with it, endometritis is rare and often indicates a predisposing factor in the patient. Acute endometritis often occurs after pregnancy components remain after an abortion or delivery or if there is a foreign body in the uterus. This condition is almost always treated after removal of pregnancy debris and treatment with appropriate antibiotics. Chronic endometritis is characterized by infiltration of lymphocytes and plasma cells into the uterus, usually following pregnancy, miscarriage, the presence of an IUD in the uterus, or PID. Genital tuberculosis occurs. The most common symptoms of this disease are vaginal bleeding and pelvic pain, and in case of clinical suspicion, culture is performed to confirm, diagnose and determine the microorganism responsible. It is often a good sign of PID. Chronic localized or extensive endometritis with squamous necrosis and metaplasia is the most common finding in women with IUDs. In some cases, the inflammation is transmitted through the fallopian tubes and leads to PID and ovarian abscesses. Antibiotics are appropriate and eliminate the underlying cause of treatment, but in very rare cases where the disease is recurrent and treated with side effects or causes side effects (such as ovarian abscesses) or the patient is unwilling to maintain fertility, hysterectomy is considered.

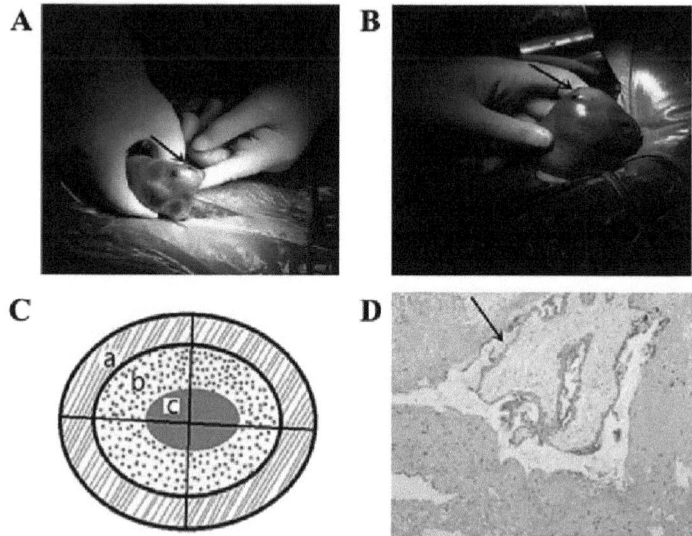

Figure 8. Lesion appearance, schema chart and pathological section

Endometriosis and Adenomyosis

Endometriosis is the presence of uterine tissue in a location other than the uterus, and adenomyosis is the replacement of islets of endometrial tissue in the uterine myometrium. Although both lesions are caused by the presence of uterine tissue in an abnormal location, they have completely different microscopic pathogenesis. In endometriosis, atopic uterine tissue is often active and undergoes structural changes. It is derived and inactivated so that in the uterine secretory phase changes corresponding to this condition are seen in only a quarter of the tissue and most of this atopic tissue has a proliferative appearance. In terms of clinical signs, both lesions cause pelvic pain associated with menstruation Which is the most important symptom of these lesions and makes it difficult to differentiate between the two according to clinical symptoms.

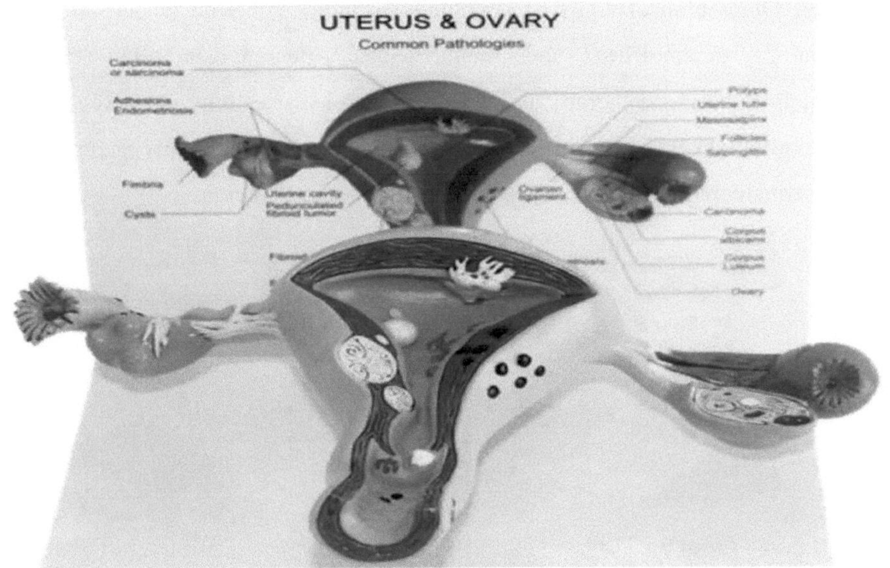

Figure 9. MASII Anatomical Uterine Model Pathology of the Uterine lesion Model Uterine Model the Odorid

Adenomyosis

The two parts of the endometrium and uterine myometrium are usually distinctly distinct from each other, but in some cases their distance is not easily seen. The distance between the myometrium and the endometrium inside the myometrium is considered as adenomyosis. The cause of these lesions is not known, but it seems that there is a direct relationship between the occurrence of this lesion and pregnancy due to the special characteristics of this lesion and its diagnosis only. It is recorded microscopically. There is disagreement about its prevalence. While pathological authorities often state the prevalence of this lesion between 15 to 20% in different obstetric and gynecological authorities, a wider range of (7 to 40) percent has been reported in a new method that has been done through multiple uterine sampling. Adenomyosis is often associated with large, globular uterus, which is always associated with the lesion due to myometrial hypertrophy. This condition may be the reason for the dangerous complication of adenomyosis, ie rupture of the uterus during pregnancy. Other clinical signs of adenomyosis include uterine tenderness, colic, pelvic pain, dysmenorrhea, and menorrhagia. Adenomyosis often responds appropriately to hormone therapy and curettage, and hysterectomy is rarely required. Therefore, although this lesion is a common finding in hysterectomy specimens, it cannot be considered an initial common indication for hysterectomy.

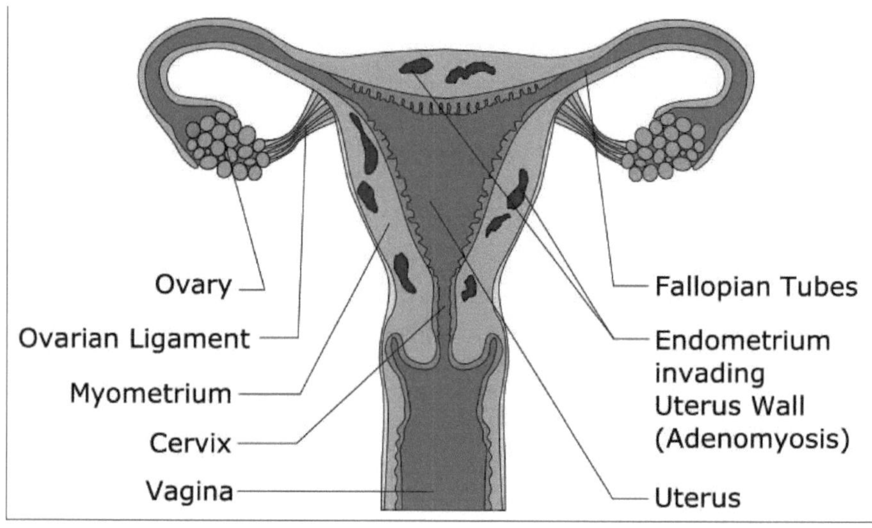

Figure 10. Adenomyosis: Causes, Symptoms and Treatment

Endometriosis

Endometriosis is found in different tissues, the most common of which are: ovaries, uterine ligaments, rectovaginal septum, pelvic peritoneum, appendix, and endometriosis. Eventually they become infertile, which is the most important complication of this disease. Since confirmation of the diagnosis of endometriosis requires surgery, there is no definitive information about its prevalence, but some sources consider 10% of all women to be close to reality, and in the United States it seems to be between 1 and 7%. There is accurate information about endometriosis-related hysterectomies, so that it was found that this lesion is responsible for only 5%

of hysterectomies and in more than 90% of cases, the preoperative diagnosis of this lesion is consistent with subsequent pathological findings.

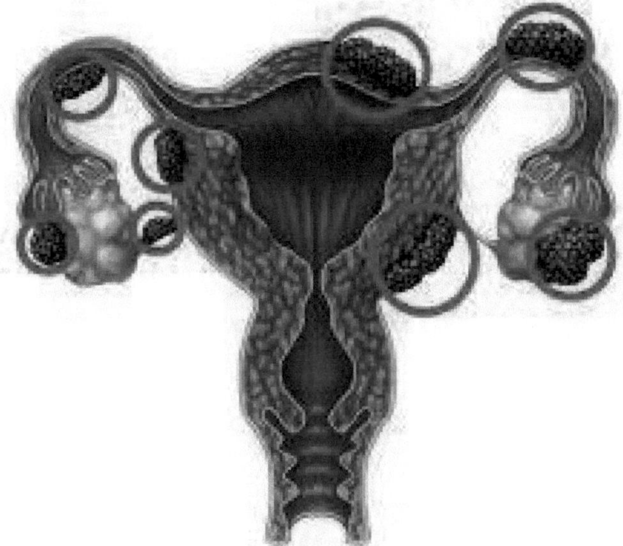

Figure 11. Endometriosis

Diagnosis of Pathology

The microscopic diagnosis of endometriosis is based on two of the following three findings:

- Existence of endometrial glands
- Presence of endometrial stroma
- Existence of homosiderin pigment

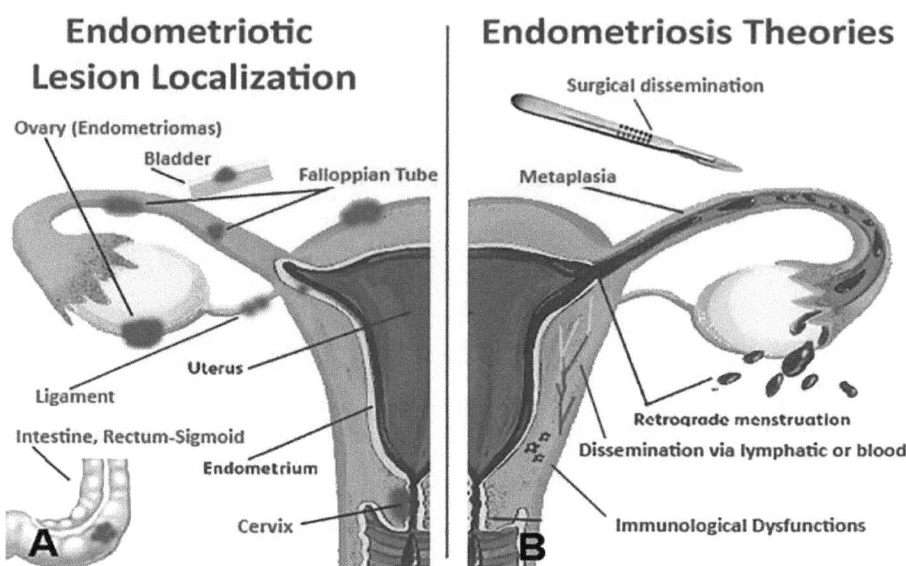

Figure 12. Frontiers | Immunological Basis of the Endometriosis: The Complement System

Endometrial Polyps

The majority of endometrial polyps are not true neoplasms and are in fact composed of limited areas of hyperplasticity with cystic glandular changes. Glandostyroma of endometrial polyps is resistant to progesterone stimulation and maintains its stability during different uterine phases. However, polyps with active and functional tissues have been reported rarely. Decisions about how to treat endometrial polyps are usually made based on the patient's clinical symptoms, the number and extent of the lesions, and the patient's physical and age status, which can include a wide range of conservative or surgical treatments.

Endometrial hyperplasia

Endometrial hyperplasia is of great importance due to the etiological association with the occurrence of DUB (as the second leading cause of DUB after non-ovulatory cycles) and the possibility of neoplastic changes associated with endometrial carcinoma. And a lack of proper progesterone activity occurs. (Unopposed strogenic effect) This condition is actually considered a major risk factor for endometrial carcinoma. Some of the conditions that cause endometrial hyperplasia due to the above conditions are recurrent non-ovulatory cycles, polycystic ovary diseases (including stein leventhal syndrome), active tumors of the ovarian granulosa cells, and ovarian granulosa and ovulation. Accurate atypia is very important in endometrial hyperplasia and is the interpretation used by the pathologist that guides the physician in choosing the appropriate treatment from periodic treatment with progestin to hysterectomy. Endometrial hyperplasia is divided into 3 types: atypical, complex It can be seen that the microscopic differentiation of these 3 types of lesions is as follows:

1. In simple types, the endometrial glands dilate and form a cystic shape, and the lining of these glands is of the ligative type with little budding and they have no future.
2. In complex types, like the simple type, the covering of proliferative glands is without atypia, but there are many budding.
3. Atypic type may occur in any of the previous two types and is distinguished from them by changes in atypicality. The importance of this type is in the high probability of malignancy in these lesions.

Endometrial Carcinoma

Endometrial carcinoma is the most invasive and common malignancy of the female genital tract in the United States and accounts for about 7% of all female genital neoplasms (except skin malignancies).

This lesion often occurs in old age, so it is very rare in people under the age of40. In 80% of cases, the lesion is discovered after menopause, and the largest group of patients is women between 55 and 65 years old.

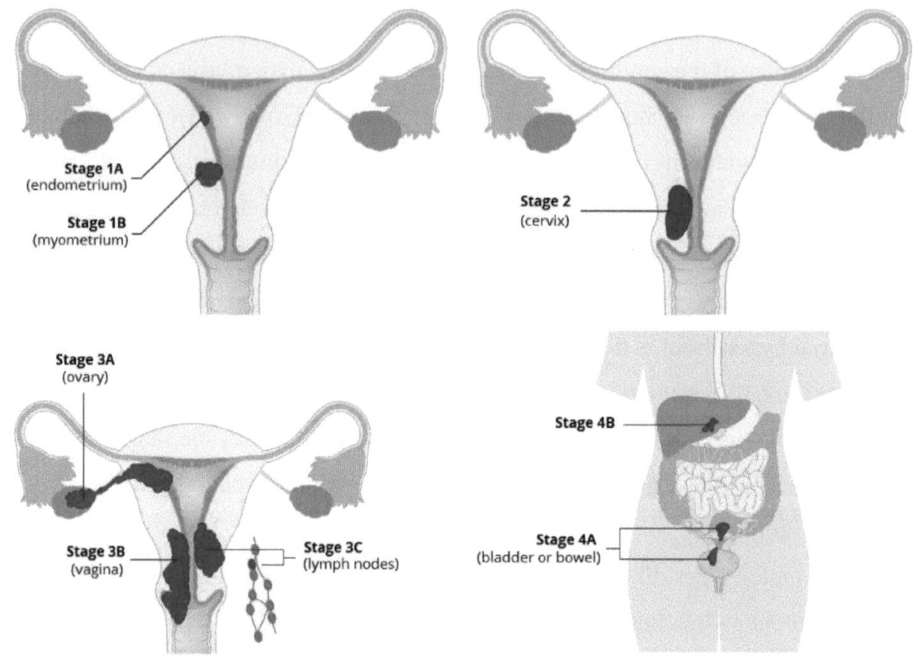

Figure 13. Endometrial Cancer

The main risk factors for endometrial carcinoma are:

I. Obesity
II. Diabetes
III. High blood pressure
IV. Absence of ovulation or ovulation disorder
V. Infertility
VI. Long-term use of estrogen hormones
VII. Tumor cells and active ovarian granulosa
VIII. Gonadal dysgenesis (Turner syndrome)
IX. Pelvic radiotherapy (radiotherapy)
X. Long-term use of tamoxifen (for the treatment of breast cancer)

Endometrial adenocarcinoma accounts for 80% of endometrial malignancies, of which 50% are differentiated (grade I), 35% are semi-differentiated (grade II), and 15% are undifferentiated (grade III).

Clinical symptoms and diagnosis

Fortunately, despite the invasiveness of endometrial carcinoma, since it often causes postmenopausal bleeding, it is quickly diagnosed and treated in the early stages. Endometrial carcinoma can remain asymptomatic for some time, but often causes abnormal bleeding, leukorrhea, and in advanced stages of uterine enlargement. If the lesion is clinically diagnosed, it should be confirmed by endometrial curettage and microscopic examination.

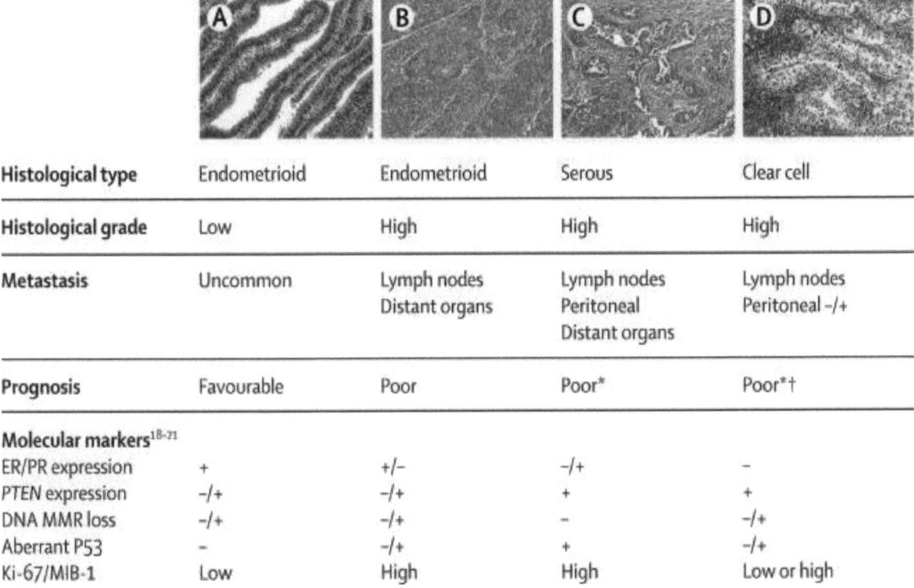

	A	B	C	D
Histological type	Endometrioid	Endometrioid	Serous	Clear cell
Histological grade	Low	High	High	High
Metastasis	Uncommon	Lymph nodes Distant organs	Lymph nodes Peritoneal Distant organs	Lymph nodes Peritoneal -/+
Prognosis	Favourable	Poor	Poor*	Poor*†
Molecular markers[18-21]				
ER/PR expression	+	+/-	-/+	-
PTEN expression	-/+	-/+	+	+
DNA MMR loss	-/+	-/+	-	-/+
Aberrant P53	-	-/+	+	-/+
Ki-67/MIB-1	Low	High	High	Low or high

Figure 14. Classification of endometrial carcinoma: more than two types

Prognosis

The prognosis of endometrial carcinoma depends to a large extent on the clinical stage (staging) and the histological grade of the lesion at the time of diagnosis.

In the United States, about 80% of patients have differentiated lesions at the time of diagnosis in clinical stage I. Surgery in stage I of the disease is associated with a survival rate of 90%, in stage II 30 to 50% and in higher stages about 20% for 5 years.

Staging of endometrial carcinoma in the FIGO system The FIGO grading system is mainly defined by the tumor growth pattern and to a lesser extent by the degree of cellular atypia.

Stage IA: Tumor confined to the endometrium

Stage IB: The lesion involves half of the myometrial wall

Stage IC: The lesion affects more than half of the myometrium

Stage IIA: Endocervical gland involvement

Stage IIIB: Cervical stromal involvement

Stage IIIA: Involvement of uterine appendages or uterine serosa or positive peritoneal cytology

Stage IIIB: Vaginal metastasis

Stage IIIC: metastasis to the pelvic or paraaortic lymph nodes

Stage IVA: Involvement of the bladder or intestinal mucosa

Stage IVB: Distant metastasis

From a diagnostic point of view, unfortunately, Pap smear test is not sufficient for proper screening of endometrial carcinoma and will be positive in only 50% of cases. The presence of normal endometrial cells in cervical cytologies may be a sign of endometrial hyperplasia or carcinoma depending on the patient's clinical condition and LMP, and is considered an indication for endometrial cytological examination by more specialized devices.

Proliferation and metastasis

The most common sites of ectopic spread are endometrial adenocarcinomas, pelvic, paraaortic lymph nodes, and ovaries. Lymph node metastasis occurs in only 5 to 25% of high-grade tumors in stage I, and in 8% of cases, endometrial carcinomas are seen at the same time as ovarian carcinoma. It will be difficult to determine if the endometrium is independent or if one is metastatic to the other. Distant metastases often occur in the lung, liver, bone, CNS, and skin, and are the most common site of recurrence after vaginal and pelvic treatment.

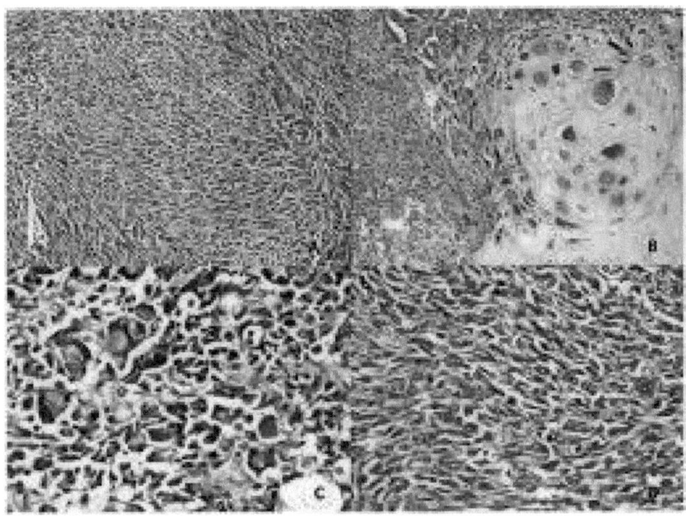

Figure 15. Primary ovarian malignant mixed mullerian tumors / carcinosarcomas: a clinico-pathological

Treatment

The most common treatment for endometrial carcinomas is a hysterectomy with bilateral salpingo-oophorectomy, which depending on the lesion can be accompanied by removal of the pelvic and paraaortic lymph nodes. Hysterectomy is performed routinely, except in some special cases, it has little therapeutic value and today the use of this method is not recommended routinely. Tumor recurrence in 50% of cases as local recurrence, in 28% of cases as distant metastasis and 21% of cases It is seen together 1-2 years after the initial treatment and local recurrences of the lesion can be successfully treated with extensive radiation therapy.

Malignant mixed mullerian tumor (n\miced mesodermal tumor)

Malignant tumors of the malignant molar are invasive and progressive neoplasms that are seen especially in older age and after menopause. These lesions often cause abnormal uterine bleeding and enlargement of the uterus. The most common site is the posterior wall of the uterine fundus. Macroscopically, these lesions are large, soft, polypoid masses that grow in the endometrium and myometrium, and in some cases protrude from the cervical opening. neuroectodermal) but due to the incidence at older ages and the lack of skin, glial and thyroid tissue components are differentiated from teratomas.

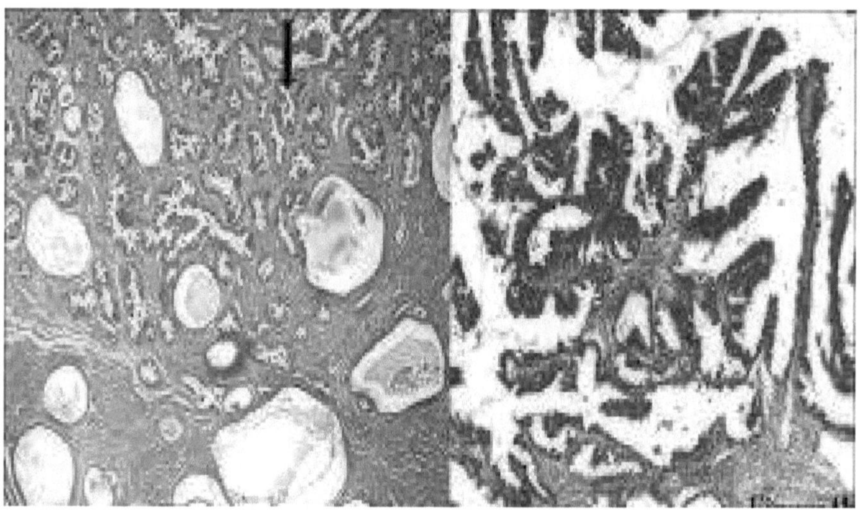

Figure 16. Malignant mixed Mullerian tumor of broad ligament with synchronous ovarian

Mixed neoplasms of mixed neoplasms are more invasive than endometrial carcinomas and are highly dilated or dilated. The prognosis of these lesions is very disappointing if they have spread outside the uterus during surgery, and only in cases where less than half of the myometrium is involved can be expected to survive properly after surgery.

Selective treatment in the case of these lesions is complete abdominal hysterectomy with bilateral removal of uterine appendages and pelvic lymphadenectomy. There is no agreement about radiotherapy and its effectiveness in the treatment of this lesion and some authorities recommend it.

Uterine leiomyome

Uterine leiomyomas are the most common pelvic tumors in women. The overall incidence of these lesions is 10% and its prevalence in the population of women over 50 years is considered to be about 40%. These lesions are often small and asymptomatic and go undiagnosed, but careful examination of hysterectomy specimens shows that uterine leiomyomas are one of the post-hysterectomy diagnoses. In a recent systematic study of 100 hysterectomies, 77 uterine leiomyoma specimens were found, 84% of which were multifocal lesions.

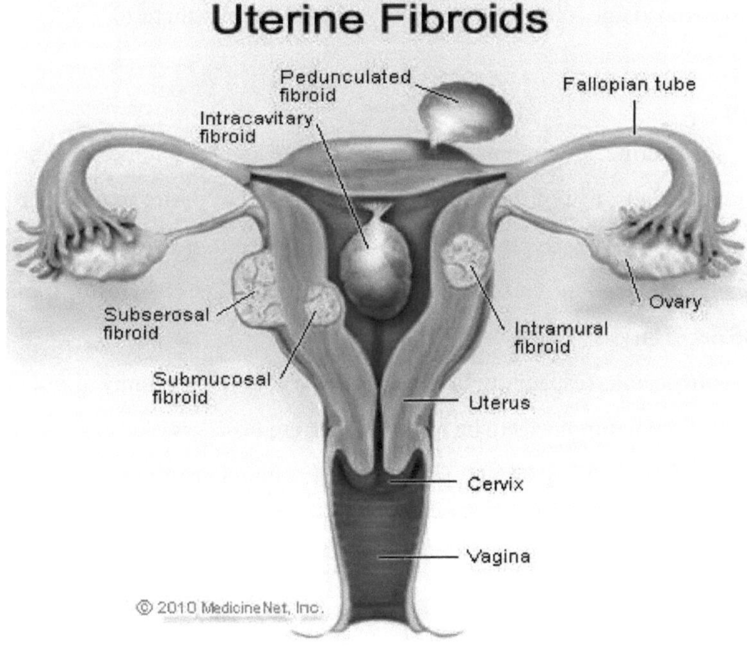

Figure 17. Uterine Fibroids: Causes, Treatment, Symptoms, Diet & Surgery

Neoplasms are benign and estrogen-dependent, so new lesions almost never develop after menopause, and previously asymptomatic lesions are not symptomatic, but rather degenerate and become calcified. The opposite happens during pregnancy, as most uterine leiomas grow larger during pregnancy and may even reach several times their pre-pregnancy size.

Signs

Uterine leiomyomas are usually divided into three types: submucosal, subserosal, and interamural, which may be symptomatic depending on their size and location. Submucosal lesions are more symptomatic than other lesions and are the most common clinical symptoms in patients with; Uterine leiomyomas include abnormal uterine bleeding, miscarriage, pelvic pain, and frequent urination. Other complications of uterine leiomyomas include inappropriate fetal presentations, uterine inertia and postpartum hemorrhage, fertility disorders, and ureteral obstruction.

Treatment

Treatment for uterine leiomyomas varies according to the number and size of the lesions, clinical signs, age of the patient, and the degree of desire to maintain fertility. Most of these lesions are asymptomatic and do not need to be removed. And is about 0.2 to 0.7 percent. Preventive surgery to prevent malignant changes in these lesions will not be necessary.

In symptomatic lesions (especially submucosal types), a hysterectomy or myomectomy is performed if the tumor needs to be removed. Limited surgery, such as myomectomy, is usually preferred for patients who wish to maintain their fertility. Uterine leiomyomas are the most common cause of hysterectomy and are responsible for 30% of cases, but today medical methods such as the use of gonadotropin-releasing hormone analogues are also used to treat these lesions and reduce patients' symptoms. There are different types of uterine leiomyomas, including atypical types with nuclear pleomorphism, large cells, and giant cells, but no necrosis is seen, and the number of mitoses in 10 strong visual fields (HPF) is less than 10.

Uterine leiomyosarcoma uterine leiomyosarcoma

Leiomyosarcomas are malignant neoplasms of the uterus that are very rare compared to leiomyomas and are seen in the older age group than leiomyomas. The mean age of patients is 54 years. Recent research has largely ruled out the possibility of these lesions from leiomyomas.

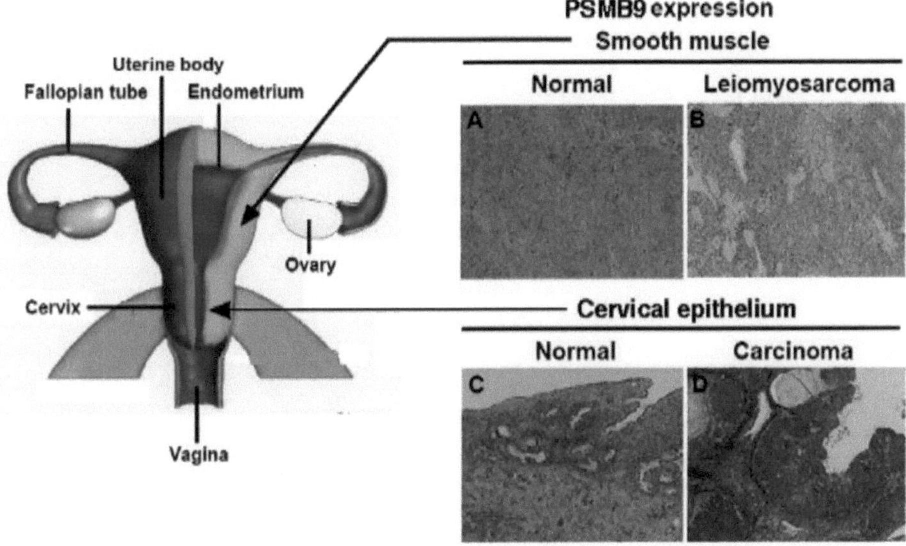

Figure 18. Molecular Pathology and Novel Clinical Therapy for Uterine Leiomyosarcoma

Elliptical and spindle-shaped cells are characterized by smooth muscle cells that can be differentiated from uterine leiomyomas due to their numerous mitotic forms. The prognosis of these tumors is more related to the normal and clinical course of the lesion. Today, the spread of this lesion to the uterus is a prognostic factor. In a credible study by Bartsich et al., Of 20 patients with uterine leiomyosarcoma who were monitored for extrauterine expansion, none survived until 29 months after diagnosis. The most common sign of malignancy in these lesions is local recurrence in the pelvic area, although distant metastases (especially to the lungs) also occur.

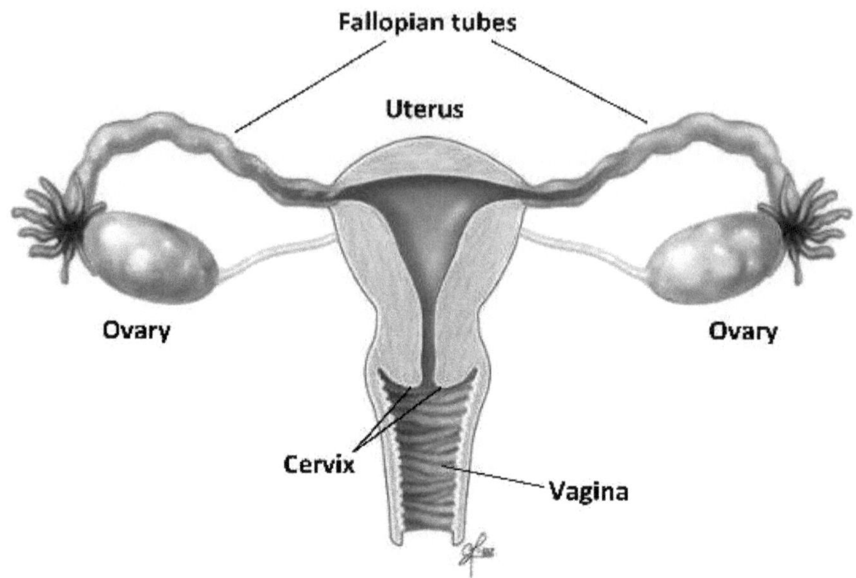

Figure 19. Uterine Sarcoma: Symptoms, Tests, Prognosis & Treatment

State the problem and the need to implement the plan

Current problem situation based on available information and data

Uterine and cervical diseases include polyps, helium endometritis, cervicitis, uterine cancer, cervical cancer, endometrial hyperplasia, endomyosis, endometriosis and leiomyosarcoma, which we will briefly review the current status of these diseases.

Polyps

Endocervical polyps are benign inflammatory tumor lesions that are seen in2.5% of women of puberty. The polyps are mostly small and these lesions need to be differentiated from more dangerous lesions due to abnormal vaginal bleeding.

Cervical metaplasia

The term squamous metaplasia is used when the squamous epithelium replaces the glandular epithelium. This finding is so common in the cervix that it is practically considered normal and occurs in almost all women of childbearing age. It is a type of cervical metaplasia.

Cervical squamous cell neoplasms

Fifty years ago, cervical carcinoma was the leading cause of death for women with cancer in most countries, but today the mortality rate for women with cervical cancer has dropped to 60 percent, followed by lung, breast, colon, and tonsil cancers. The ovaries, lymph nodes, and blood are in eighth place.

Cervical squamous cell carcinoma (SCC)

Despite the reduction in SCC mortality, this lesion is still the most common female genital malignancy in most parts of the world. SCC occurs at any age from20 to old age, but the most common age of onset of these invasive lesions is 40 to 45 years. Is 30 years old and in high-grade precancerous lesions. Today, due to the use of screening methods and diagnosis and treatment of these lesions is being reduced.

Other cervical carcinomas

Adenocarcinomas, adenosquamous carcinoma, Clearcell careinum, and undifferentiated carcinoma together account for 25% of all cervical cancer lesions. Cervical adenocarcinoma accounts for 5-15% of the total work of cervical sinuses.

Endometritis

Unlike cervicitis, which is a common and insignificant finding, due to the protective role of the cervix and the anatomical condition of the uterus associated with it, endometritis rarely occurs and often indicates a predisposing background in the patient. Acute endometritis often occurs after pregnancy components remain after abortion or delivery or the presence of a foreign body in the uterus. Chronic endometritis is characterized by lymphocyte and plasma cell infiltration into the uterus.

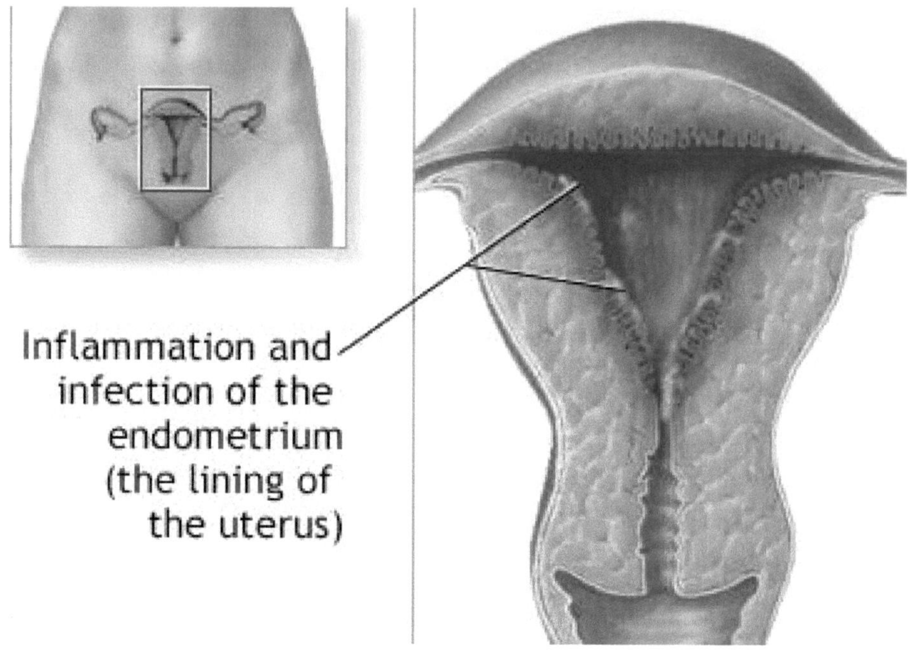

Figure 20. Endometritis Information

Endometriosis

Endometriosis is the presence of uterine tissue in a place other than the uterus. In terms of clinical signs, the lesion causes pelvic pain associated with menstruation, which is the most important symptom of this lesion. Endometriosis is the most common cause of hospitalization in women aged 15 to 45 years and 30-40% of patients with this lesion eventually become infertile, which is the most important complication of this lesion.

Adenomyosis

Endometrial basal invasion of the myometrium leads to the uterus often becoming large and more or less global in appearance. Pathologists often state that the prevalence of this lesion is between 15 and 20%.

Endometrial hyperplasia

Endometrial hyperplasia is of great importance due to the etiological association with the occurrence of DUB and the possibility of neoplastic changes associated with endometrial carcinoma. Endometrial hyperplasia includes simple, complex, and atypical types, in which the atypical type has a high risk of malignancy.

Endometrial carcinoma

It is the most invasive and common female genital malignancy in the United States and accounts for about 7% of all female genital neoplasms (except skin malignancy). This lesion often occurs in old age so that it is very rare under the age of 40 and in 80% of cases the lesion is discovered after menopause and the largest group of patients are 55-65 years old. Endometrial adenocarcinoma accounts for 80% of endometrial malignancies, of which 50% are differentiated,35% are semi-differentiated, and 15% are not differentiated.

Uterine leiomyomas

The most common pelvic tumors are women, the overall incidence of these lesions is 10% and its prevalence in the population of women over 50 years is40%. Leiomyum includes subcortical, subserosal, and intracellular types that may be marked depending on size and location.

Lumium of uterine sarcoma

Malignant neoplasms of the uterus are very rare compared to leiomyoma and are seen in the older age group than leiomyoma, so the average age is 54 years.

Health-economic-social-political effects of the current form

Due to the wide range of uterine and cervical diseases in women, a significant percentage of women experience these diseases at some point in their lives. Many of these diseases have a direct and adverse effect on individual, social, economic and health activities. Early diagnosis and diagnosis and prevention of disease progression have an effective role in reducing or eliminating these adverse effects and due to the high prevalence of these diseases, examination from both clinical and pathological perspectives is important.

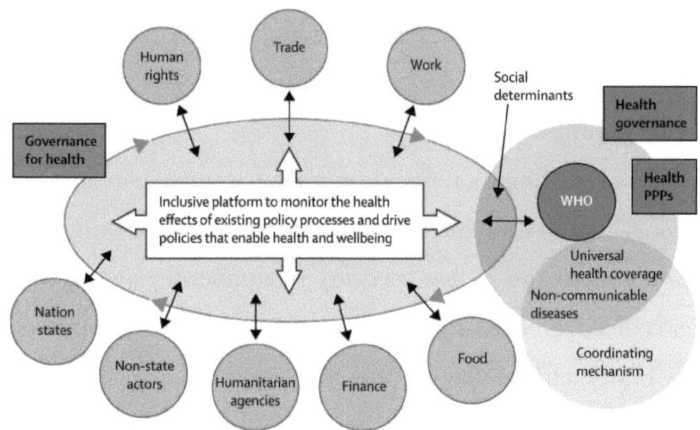

Figure 21. The political origins of health inequity: prospects for change

For example, today, hysterectomy is the second most common surgery in most countries after cesarean section due to diseases of the female genital tract. One in three American women under the age of 60 has undergone this operation and the cost of performing this number of operations. Hysterectomy costs more than $ 50 billion a year. These diseases have harmful effects on the individual, society and economy.

The economic, social and cultural status of these diseases can be seen at all levels of society, including advanced and developing societies. It has also been reported that the prognosis of these diseases is weaker in less developed societies. And has a better prognosis in developed societies due to diagnosis, treatment, and screening, and given the wider medical possibilities.

Factors influencing and related to the topic

Due to the importance of the issue, the role of risk factors in these patients (age, race, infection, pregnancy) should be identified and identified to eliminate these factors to reduce the prevalence of these patients. The female reproductive system is prone to certain pathological lesions due to its anatomical condition and the impact of physiological changes such as menstrual cycles and gestational periods. It is very important. In the case of cervical squamous cell neoplasms, studies show that the incidence of this lesion is significantly related to a person's sexual activity, so that it is almost never seen among nuns, and the main risk factors for this lesion are:

1. The young age of the person at the beginning of sexual activity
2. Having multiple sexual partners
3. Having a male sexual partner who has been in a relationship with multiple sexual partners.

In this regard, human papillomavirus (HPV) is considered as the most important factor in the oncogenicity of cervical lesions and infection with 18, 16 and 13 types is more risky and causes high-grade lesions, about 75% of women during life. They become infected with the virus, which accounts for only 10% of intraepithelial neoplasms (CINs), and a small percentage of 1.3%) of invasive carcinoma.

Other risk factors include smoking, multiparous, nutritional factors, and immune system changes for cervical neoplasms.

- ✓ Other cervical cancers, which account for 25 percent of all cervical cancer lesions, include factors such as race, which is more prevalent in Jews, and HPV18 and diethyl acetylbastrol during pregnancy.
- ✓ It is now known that endometrial hyperplasia is caused by strong and long-term estrogenic stimuli and lack of proper progesterone activity. This condition is actually considered a major risk factor for endometrial carcinoma. Other contributing factors include repeated non-ovulatory cycles, polycystic ovary diseases, and active ovarian granulosa cell tumors.

Risk factors for endometrial carcinoma include:

I. Obesity
II. Diabetes
III. Blood pressure
IV. No ovulation or ovulation disorder
V. Infertility

VI. Pelvic radiation therapy

VII. Long-term use of estrogen hormones

VIII. Gonadal dysgenesis (Turner syndrome)

IX. A long-acting reagent of tamoxifen

In the case of uterine leiomyomas, a strong association can be made between these diseases and estrogen. Therefore, these lesions almost never occur after menopause and the previous lesions are also analyzed.

What steps are currently being taken or are being taken to resolve the issue

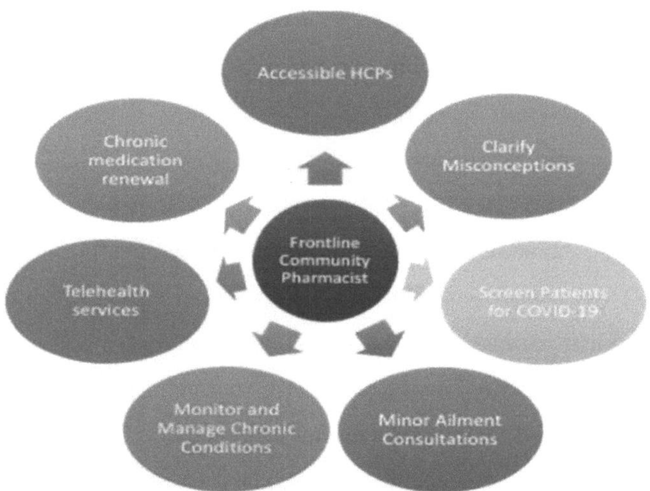

Figure 22. Pharmacists and COVID-19

Given the importance of uterine and cervical patients, these diseases should be given more attention and research, and research that has been done before and even now under study and progress confirms this importance.

- ✓ Reducing the prevalence of neck cancers is due to the invention of Pap smears and other new research methods and their widespread use are recent pains, and to reduce the adverse effects of this disease, measures are taken including hysterectomy and conservative surgeries.

- ✓ For endometritis, desirable and approved methods such as accurate administration of antibiotics and elimination of underlying factors are performed, and if these methods fail or the person does not want to become pregnant, a hysterectomy can be used.
- ✓ For endometriosis diseases, because more than 90% of cases with pathological findings are consistent with the definitive diagnosis, unnecessary hysterectomy can be reduced by pathological examination.
- ✓ In many cases of endometrial hyperplasia, which presents with spotting and bleeding, can be examined and diagnosed by biopsy or D & C, and if diagnosed by progesterone treatments and follow-up to treat the lesions, and if no response. Encourage treatment with either atypical hyperplasia or unwillingness to conceive.
- ✓ In the case of endometrial carcinomas, hysterectomy with bilateral resection of the uterine appendages, which, depending on the lesion, can be accompanied by removal of the pelvic and paraaortic lymph nodes. Recent research has shown that radiotherapy, which has been commonly performed with voice hysterectomy until recent years, has little therapeutic value except in special cases.
- ✓ Most uterine leiomas are asymptomatic and have a low risk of malignancy and do not need to be removed, and preventive surgery is not necessary to prevent malignant changes in these lesions.
- ✓ Cervical polyps require differentiation from more dangerous lesions due to abnormal vaginal bleeding. The surface epithelium of these lesions is often metaplasia, but the incidence of cervical intraepithelial neoplasia (CIN) is not higher than in other areas of the cervix. Cases with simple curettage or removal of polyps with surgical methods can eliminate complications.

What is your suggestion for solving the problem based on the above findings?
Based on the above findings, it is clear that women after puberty, due to anatomical and physiological issues, the genitals are exposed to a variety of benign to malignant

diseases. Therefore, it is suggested that treatment measures be taken by screening and diagnosis studies and according to the findings and risk factors that threaten them. It is recommended that annual Pap smear examinations be performed to carefully and thoroughly treat infections that occur during life, and to evaluate chronic endometritis if mechanical contraceptives such as the diaphragm and IUD are used. If the person has AUB, a complete biopsy and examination should be performed and patients with atypical or refractory hyperplasia may be recommended for hysterectomy.

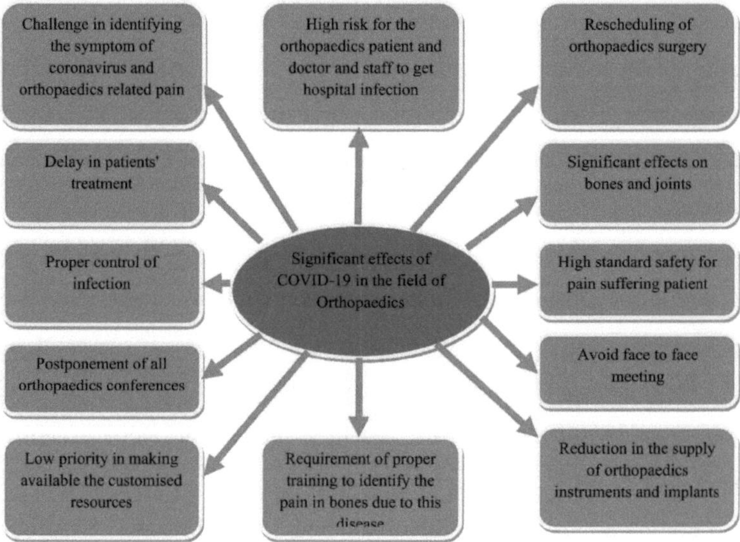

Figure 23. Effects of COVID-19 pandemic in the field of orthopaedics

Chapter II

Background and background of the research

In a study by Baryan Hunry and Lina Blony, 273 pathological slides were examined for pathological lesions of the uterus and cervix. The most common lesions in this study were as follows:

Chronic cervicitis 26.4%, uterine leiomyoma 15.8%, adenomyosis 14.4%, cervical polyps 13.1%, endometrial polyps 9%, endometrial carcinoma 7.1%, endometrial hyperplasia 6.3% and endometriosis 5.1 % have been. In this study, the prevalence of uterine and cervical cancers, endometrial adenocarcinoma was 64.3%, SCC cervix was 21.6% and leiomyosarcoma was 8.3%. In another study by Michel Charls, the most common age for uterine involvement with malignant tumors is 50-60 years and cervical involvement is 45-55 years. The prevalence of endometrial polyps and cervical polyps decreases with age, and the frequency of cervical and endometrial cancer increases with age, with 75% being discovered after menopause, and squamous metaplasia is so common in women of childbearing age that it is so common.

Handley examined the role of female circumcision in the development of cervical and cervical cancers, which had a lower incidence of cancer than others. Kessler said women whose husbands had previously had wives with cervical cancer had a higher risk of developing cancer.

Rowls, Josseg et al. Found an association between HSV type 2 and cervical cancer. In 1980, it was discovered that DNA and HPV were found in these lesions, and that the presence of HPV infection would be a major risk factor for cervical cancer and CIN. The role of tobacco use, nutritional factors and OCP has also been proven. Cervical carcinoma is the second most common cancer in women, and it is more common in communities with low economic status and in women who have had sex at a younger age and in greater numbers.

Eddy, Davidm in an article entitled Cervical Cancer Screening in 1998 presents a collection of information obtained from articles and studies of different people about the prevalence and contributing factors of cervical cancer. In this article, the incidence of cervical cancer "130 per 100,000" in the age of 25-35 years has been reported. Which increases to "200 per 100,000" at the age of 50 and states that this prevalence is related to women who have undergone a screening program.

Herman-P and Gaspard-u in a study of women aged 30-75 years and a hysterectomy performed on all of these individuals, it was found that inflammatory lesions were most common in middle-aged people, and that these lesions were significantly reduced at younger and older ages. And has decreased to less than 20% and malignant lesions of the uterus and cervix have increased significantly in older ages, which is 12 times more in those over 50 years old than in those under 50 years old.

According to Ms. Shamila Vahidi's dissertation in2000, the most important risk factors for cervical cancer are the onset of sexual activity, especially under the age of 20, young age during the first pregnancy, having multiple sexual partners, and instability in marriage and intimacy with high-risk men. Frequency of sexual intercourse, menstrual patterns, number of pregnancies and male circumcision are not important factors. Immunosuppressive treatments and pelvic radiotherapy are among the underlying factors.

As can be seen in the table, the most common lesion in this study is chronic service, which is about 34%, followed by uterine leiomyoma with 18.2% and adenomyosis with 12.4%. The rarest leiomyosarcoma lesion is SCC cervix, endometritis with a frequency of 0.3%. Also, four chronic cervical lesions, uterine leiomyoma, adenomyosis and cervical polyps were present in 120 cases as concomitant lesions.

Table 1. Frequency of various pathological lesions of the uterus and cervix

Relative cumulative frequency	Relative abundance	Absolute abundance	Pathology
34	34	244	Chronic service
52/2	18/2	131	Lymioma of the uterus
46/6	12/4	89	Adenomyosis
73/3	8/7	63	Chronic service and uterine leiomyoma
78/7	5/4	39	Chronic service and adenomyosis

81/2	2/5	18	Chronic service and cervical polyps
89	7/8	56	Polyps of the cervix
92/3	3/3	24	Endometrial polyps
93/7	1/4	10	Atrophic endometrium
95/1	1/4	10	Mol Hidati Form
96/5	1/4	10	Endometrial carcinoma
97/3	0/8	6	Endometrial hyperplasia
97/9	0/6	4	Heterogeneous endometrium
98/5	0/6	4	Endometriosis
99/1	0/6	4	Myometritis
99/4	0/3	2	Endometritis
99/7	0/3	2	SCC Cervix
100	0/3	2	Leiomyosarcoma

Table 2: Frequency of pathological lesions of uterus and cervix by age groups

Total		Above 70 years		70-56 years		55-41 years		40-25 years		Under 25 years		Pathology
Relative	Absolute	Relative	Absolute	Relative	Absolute	Relative	Absolute	Relative	Absolute	Relative	Absolute	
100	244	2/9	7	4/5	11	68/4	167	23/8	58	0/4	1	Chronic service
100	131	0/8	1	3/8	5	64/1	84	28/3	37	3	4	Lymioma of the uterus
100	89	1/1	1	4/5	4	83/2	74	10/1	9	1/1	1	Adenomyosis
100	63	1/6	1	3/2	2	61/9	39	31/7	20	1/6	1	Chronic service and uterine leiomyoma
100	39	0	0	5/1	2	77	30	15/4	6	2/5	1	Chronic service and adenomyosis
100	18	5/5	1	5/5	1	66/7	12	22/3	4	0	0	Chronic service and cervical polyps

100	56	7/1	4	9	5	60/7	34	23/2	13	0	0	Polyps of the cervix
100	24	0	0	0	0	83/3	20	16/7	4	0	0	Endometrial polyps
100	10	0	0	20	2	80	8	0	0	0	0	Atrophic endometrium
100	10	0	0	20	2	20	2	0	0	60	6	Hydatid model
100	10	40	4	0	0	40	4	20	2	0	0	Endometrial carcinoma
100	4	0	0	0	0	100	4	0	0	0	0	Heterogeneous endometrium
100	6	0	0	33/3	2	66/7	4	0	0	0	0	Endometrial hyperplasia
100	4	0	0	0	0	100	4	0	0	0	0	Endometriosis
100	4	0	0	50	2	0	0	0	0	50	2	Myometritis
100	2	0	0	0	0	0	0	100	2	0	0	Endometritis
100	2	100	2	0	0	0	0	0	0	0	0	SCC Cervix
100	2	50	1	50	1	0	0	0	0	0	0	Leiomyosarcoma

The following results are obtained from this table:

I. The most common age of onset of pathological lesions of the uterus and cervix in this study was 41-55 years with 486 cases with a frequency of about 69% and then 25-40 years with 155 cases with a frequency of about 21%. The lowest prevalence of lesions was under 25 years of age with 16 cases with a frequency of 2%.

II. In the case of malignant lesions, which includes a total of 14 cases, 50% of cases are over the age of 70, and no malignancies have been reported under the age of 25.

The mean age of the subjects was estimated to be 51.7 years, which is similar to the mean age mentioned in reputable medical books and research articles conducted in other countries, which is stated as 52.2 years on average.

I. It should be noted that the results of this study were obtained in the study of samples sent to the pathology department of hospitals and the samples were not selected randomly, so the statistics provided for each of the pathological lesions cannot be completely equivalent. He considered the absolute frequency of these lesions in the society.

II. The study of the age prevalence of lesions in general shows that the largest group of patients with pathological lesions of the uterus and cervix are women 40 to 55 years old, followed by women 25 to 40 years old and 55 to 70 years old in the second and third ranks. The problem indicates the high prevalence of various pathological lesions in women of reproductive age (especially 25 to 55 years).

III. The study of the prevalence of lesions in general shows that the chronic cervix is the largest group of patients with uterine and cervical lesions, followed by leiomyoma and adenomyosis, and SCC cervix, endometritis, myometritis, leiomyosarcoma, endometriosis, respectively. Prevalence is included in this group.

IV. In this study, all patients' spouses were circumcised before marriage, so there is a clear difference between the study group and other groups in other countries, especially in Western countries where the majority of wives of women with cancer and precancerous lesions were not circumcised. he ate.

V. The significant low number of cervical neoplasms in this study is due to the lack of prevalence of risk factors for this cancer in Iran, which is confirmed by some evidence such as Iranian women adhere to health and moral principles, the generality of circumcision in Iranian men and possibly The protective effect is genetic.

VI. In this study, the mean age of patients with malignant lesions was 51.4, which is 7/6 years different from the average age of 59 years related to global statistics. The difference can be the limited number of patients in this study.

VII. It seems necessary to mention a few points from the book and the hatred of women and compare it with the results of this research.

✓ Uterine polyps, which include single or multiple lesions, with or without stems due to overgrowth of glands and endometrial stroma, are more common in women 40 to 50 years old. In this study, it was about 70% in40-50-year-olds. It is close to the statistics of the Danforth book.

- ✓ Endometrial carcinoma is the most common malignancy of the genital tract, which was also the case in the study, but the age of 50-65 years is the most common age in the book Danforth and Robbins pathology, but in this study between the ages of 40-55 and over 70 years. Most cases of endometrial carcinoma have been reported, which may be due to the small number of samples in this study.
- ✓ Uterine marcoma is the most malignant uterine tumor and they are very rare. In this study, there were 2 cases of leiomyosarcoma that were reported over the age of 55, and another reason could be the small number of samples examined.
- ✓ In the case of adenomyosis, as mentioned in the Danforth book, the most common classic symptom is menorrhagia, the majority of which are symptomatic in women aged 35-50 years, which is consistent with the statistics of our study (ages 40-55).
- ✓ Leiomyum is more common in black women and its prevalence increases in the reproductive years. It is rare before menarche and decreases in size after menarche. Intensity has decreased.
- ✓ Among 90-95% of women who have given birth, there is evidence of chronic service. In this study, about 85% of the subjects in the age group of 25-50 years had chronic service.

VIII. According to Robins's pathology, about 85 to 90% of invasive cervical carcinomas are SCCs, and the majority of them are adenocarcinomas. In this study, we had 2 cases of cervical carcinoma, both of which included SCCs. It becomes.

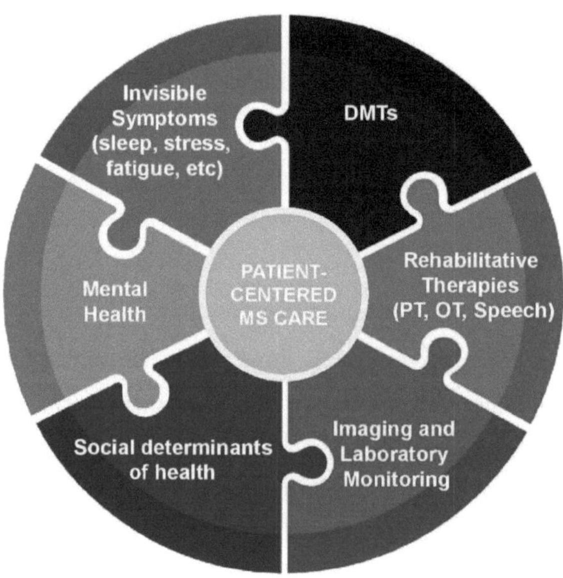

Figure 24. Pandemic forward: Lessons learned and expert perspectives on multiple sclerosis care

Chapter III

Things to Do Before Trying to Conceive

If you and your spouse are planning to have a baby, just think for a few seconds and hold for at least a month or two. In order to have a better chance of having a healthier pregnancy and a healthier baby, you need to consider a few important things before any action. The following items can help you in this regard.

Provide the body with folic acid

Even if you decide to have a balanced diet, it is very difficult to get all the nutrients you need from food alone, and this is the only thing you do not need to save. By consuming 400 micrograms of folic acid a day for at least one month before pregnancy and during the first trimester of pregnancy, you can prevent a 70% chance of having a defective child. You can also get folic acid supplements from pharmacies or take regular or prenatal multivitamins. If you are taking a multivitamin, make sure it does not contain more than the daily allowance (about 770 micrograms) of vitamin A unless it is completely in beta-carotene form. Excessive consumption of a certain type of vitamin A can lead to birth defects (congenital). If you do not know what to take, you can consult a health consultant (doctor) to prescribe a supplement.

Avoid going to parties or taking any drugs or alcohol

If you are smoking or taking medication, it is time to quit. Because some drugs stay in your body system even after they have stopped working. Numerous studies have shown that smoking and drug use can lead to miscarriage, premature birth, and low birth weight babies. In addition, research shows that any consumption of tobacco can affect fertility and reduce sperm count. In fact, some studies have shown that even cigarette smoke can affect a woman's chances of getting pregnant. Alcohol consumption can also affect pregnancy. So, the best idea is to avoid it altogether.

Avoid caffeine

Research shows that consuming too much caffeine can reduce your ability to absorb iron, which is what you need most for pregnancy, increasing your risk of stillbirth. As a result, you should stop consuming tea, coffee and cola (Pepsi, cola, Coca-Cola, etc.).

If this causes you a headache or you are so used to it that you cannot quit, you can be content with one cup a day. Most experts believe that this amount (one cup per day) may be appropriate. Instead of consuming caffeine, you can find a better alternative and consume it with milk, this will also make the calcium in milk more useful for you.

Control your weight

If you are at a healthy weight, pregnancy will be easier for you. Studies have shown that women with a body mass index (BMI) of less than 20 or more than 30 will have more problems with pregnancy. Therefore, it is better to increase your BMI between 20 and 30 before pregnancy.

Losing or gaining weight during pregnancy will help you if you do not have a healthy (proper) weight. Talk to your doctor about the best way to achieve the right weight.

Fill your refrigerator with healthy foods

Even if you do not have proper nutrition to have a healthy pregnancy, you should act now and provide the nutrients your body needs. Try to eat at least two cups of fruits and two and a half cups of vegetables daily, as well as plenty of whole grains and foods that are high in calcium, including milk, orange juice, calcium and yogurt. If you eat a lot of fish, it is better to control your consumption. Although fish is a very good source of protein, but some special types such as sharks, swordfish, etc. contain large amounts of methyl mercury, a large amount of which can be dangerous for the development of the child's brain. Because mercury accumulates in the body and stays there for more than a year, it is best to avoid fish high in mercury when you are planning to become pregnant. Instead, eat two servings of low-mercury fish a week.

Choose a suitable exercise program for yourself and follow it

Start a health plan and move on seriously, you will have a healthy and rewarding physical reward for pregnancy. A health exercise program includes 60 minutes of exercise on most days of the week, including walking, cycling and weightlifting. To increase flexibility, add exercises such as daily stretching or yoga, so you will have a more appropriate program. When you are pregnant, keep in mind that these activities are not an obstacle, and sometimes it is even recommended that you do exercise.

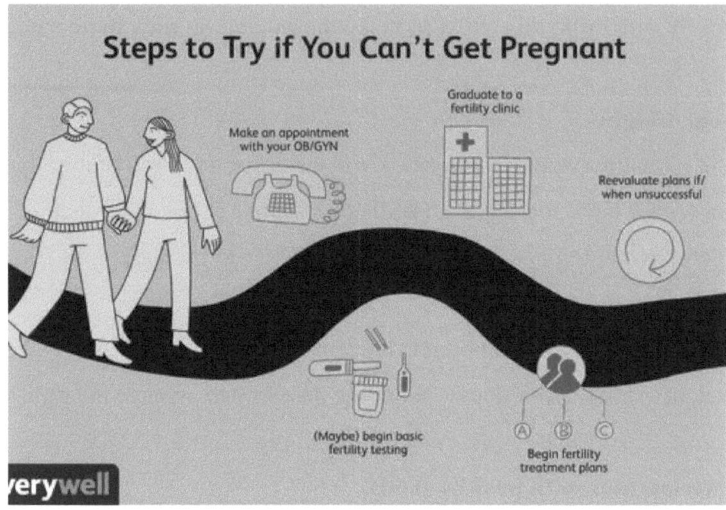

Figure 25. What to Do When You Can't Get Pregnant

See a dentist

Do not forget that when you are pregnant or planning to become pregnant, you should pay more attention to your health. There is growing evidence that periodontitis (infection of the gums), a bacterial infection that affects the gums and protective bones of the teeth, can lead to premature births or low birth weight babies. An extensive study has shown that pregnant women with periodontitis (gum infection) are seven times more likely to give birth to a premature baby. According to another study, there is a link between gum disease and an increased risk of preeclampsia, a complication of pregnancy problems with signs and symptoms such as high blood pressure, fluid retention (urine) and the presence of protein in the urine. Worse, hormonal changes during pregnancy can make you more susceptible to gum disease. Increased levels of estrogen and progesterone cause the gums to act differently against the bacteria in plaque, causing the gums to swell, bleed and become vulnerable. The good news I can give you is that women who take care of their oral health before pregnancy will not have such side effects during pregnancy. If you have not seen a dentist in the last six months, be sure to see your dentist to check your teeth and scaling.

Check the medical records of your families (male and female)

It's a good idea for you and your spouse to check on your family's health history as well, so you can ask your parents, siblings and other relatives about it. The most important thing to ask is if there are any genetic problems or disorders in the family. Or chromosomes such as Down syndrome, sickle cell disease, cystic fibrosis, Tay-Sachs disease, or blood disorders. You may also need to check with relatives if anyone has had a mental retardation or other developmental disorder and if there are any anatomical birth defects such as heart or nerve problems. Your doctor may also ask you a series of questions, and your answers will help him or her perform genetic tests on you and your partner before anything else is needed.

Plan for examination and counseling before pregnancy

You do not need to think about a midwife or obstetrician right now, but you should have a general examination. Your doctor may ask you questions about your personal and family medical history, your current state of health, and the medications you are taking. Some medications, such as Accutane, which is a prescription medication for acne, store your body fat and last for months. In addition to reviewing your diet, weight, exercise, and prescribing appropriate prenatal vitamins, your doctor will consider the following: Examine your immune system, test, and control your immunity to childhood illnesses such as rubella, syphilis, and more. Also answer your questions. Some couples insist on having genetic tests to be surer.

Consider the time of ovulation

Some women worry about getting pregnant and leave everything to chance. Others are more calculated and remember the time of ovulation. If you want to be more precise, you should note the basal body temperature and changes in the lining of the uterus. Keeping track of these symptoms will help you determine when you are ovulating. To get a more accurate temperature, you should measure your temperature early in the morning before getting out of bed with a basal thermometer available at drugstores and children's stores. Ovulation can also be detected with the help of ovulation prediction kits by detecting hormones in the urine, or changes in chloride in saliva or on the skin. These kits are also available in pharmacies and children's stores.

How to Get Pregnant
Learning the best ways to get pregnant can help couples approach the baby-making process with a more productive and less stressful mindset.
BEST TIME TO GET PREGNANT
Estimate ovulation
Track the cycles
JANUARY
Menstrual cycle
BEST WAY TO GET PREGNANT
Have frequent sex
Make sex appealing
ADDITIONAL TIPS TO CONCEIVE
Keep a healthy diet
Stay physically active
Take fertility supplements
Quit addictions

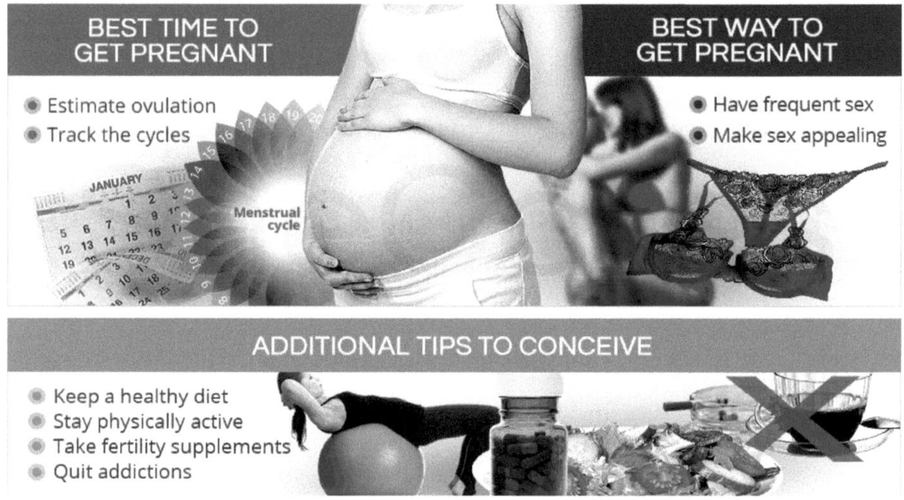

Figure 26. How to Get Pregnant: Top Tips to Conceive

Contact insurance centers

You have more than nine months to plan for hospital expenses and baby expenses. The first thing you need to do is contact the insurance companies. Thoroughly review and see what services they offer and what they cover. If you have a special midwife or doctor for you, check out her program and see how much it will cost. Find out what is exempt from insurance and what is covered by insurance in the field of prenatal examinations and tests. You may have to save some money because of the high costs so that you do not face staggering costs during pregnancy and childbirth. If you are one of those people who are not covered by any insurance, it is better to go to the insurance centers of your city or place right now and choose the most suitable one.

Meet with a financial advisor

See for yourself what to do with this rate of inflation. But do not be afraid, from now on you can save only 50 or 100 thousand Tomans per month, you can provide the best things for your child even until university. You can talk to a financial advisor about how to save.

Be aware of your mental health

According to psychologists, women who suffer from depression are twice as likely as others to have reproductive complications and problems. If someone is clinically depressed, this person can hardly take care of himself / herself, let alone have a child. From an evolutionary point of view, pregnancy is very difficult for depressed women. Psychologists believe that all women, especially those with a history of individual or family depression. They should have a mental health test before pregnancy.

If you experience symptoms of depression such as decreased interest or enjoyment in things you used to enjoy, changes in appetite, changes in sleep patterns, decreased energy, feelings of hopelessness and worthlessness, ask your doctor to refer you to a Refer to a specialist or psychologist. If treatment is needed, your psychiatrist will help you take antidepressant medication that is not harmful to you during pregnancy. You can also try stress-relieving techniques such as yoga and meditation, which researchers recommend for pregnant women with depression and stress.

Avoid infection

When you are planning to get pregnant, you need to protect yourself from all kinds of infections and diseases, especially those that harm your baby. You should also avoid foods such as unpasteurized cheese and other unpasteurized dairy products, packaged foods and meats, poultry, and raw fish. Because such foods can store dangerous bacteria that lead to diseases such as listeriosis and .... Be sure to wash your hands clean before cooking and when eating and make sure your refrigerator temperature is between 35- and 40-degrees Fahrenheit (2 and 4 degrees Celsius) and your freezer is below zero to -18 degrees Celsius. So that your food does not spoil. Finally, it is better to use gloves when digging the garden or planting, and also when replacing the trash, etc.

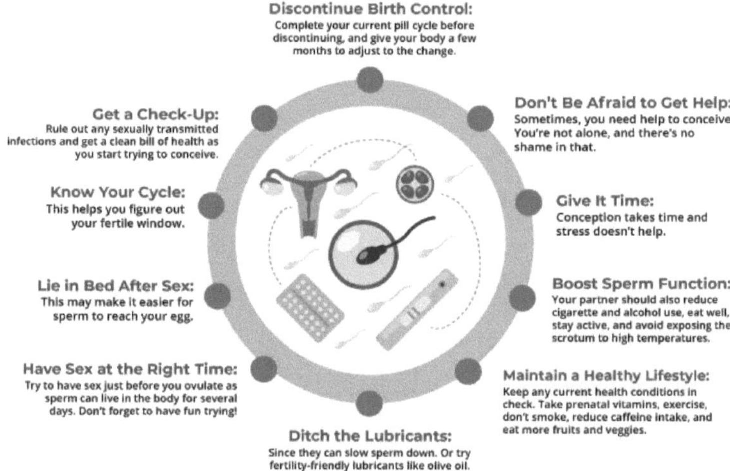

Figure 27. How to Get Pregnant Fast (10 Tips for Faster Conception)

Eliminate your environmental and work environment hazards

Some things can be dangerous for you and your baby. If you are exposed to chemicals or radiation on a daily basis, you should make changes to your work before becoming pregnant. Also keep in mind that some detergents, pesticides, solutions and even drinking water from old pipes can be dangerous for your baby's growth. Talk to your doctor about your work and the environment so that, if possible, steps can be taken to eliminate and reduce the risk factors for the workplace and home.

Think more about your decision (intention to get pregnant)

Before deciding to have children, you and your spouse need to define your purpose and see if you are ready to take on this great responsibility. Here are some key questions to keep in mind:

Are you both ready to become parents?

If you have religious differences, discuss it first and see how it will affect your child.

Have you thought about the responsibilities of raising a child and balancing work and family?

Are you ready to meet your child's needs?

Are you willing to give up sleeping and resting on your holidays?

Are you ready to take care of your child, in times when you cannot take care of him / yourself?

Tell a friend

Although motherhood is exciting, it can also be stressful at times. Trust a close friend in addition to your spouse. She can support you in times of trouble, especially when your spouse is not there.

Beware of frequent deliveries. (Prevention to control childbirth)

Although contraception is easy for many to discard, keep in mind that contraception is not easy and requires more careful planning.

For example, if you are taking birth control pills, it is best to take a whole pack to avoid irregular bleeding. It may take several months for menstruation to return to normal, but many become pregnant within a month of stopping the pill. The same is true for other contraceptives and devices such as IUDs, etc. It may take up to one year for ovulation to resume, even after discontinuation of this method, even if the period is regulated much sooner and returns to normal.

For the last time, safely do the exciting activities and tasks that you like

Before getting pregnant for the last time, do the things you love that are dangerous for pregnancy, such as horseback riding, air train riding, sauna, etc. Because it is not clear when you can do such things again.

What are the ways to prevent HIV transmission?

In summary, HIV prevention measures can be divided into three categories:

Prevention of opportunistic infections in HIV-infected people.

Prevention of HIV infection in high-risk groups.

Prevention of HIV infection in the general population.

1- Considering that the most important consequence of HIV infection is the occurrence of opportunistic infections, therefore, the occurrence of these infections in HIV-positive people should be avoided as much as possible. Two things can be done for this purpose:

A- Drug prevention: In the case of some opportunistic infections, such as tuberculosis, medications can be used to prevent their occurrence in HIV-positive and HIV-infected people.

B- Vaccination: By vaccinating HIV-positive people, infections such as pneumonia, diphtheria and tetanus, influenza, etc. can be prevented.

2- Some individuals and groups, such as injecting drug users, health care workers, infants born to HIV-positive mothers, people with sexually transmitted infections, and people with high-risk sexual behaviors, are at high risk for HIV infection. Therefore, more attention should be paid to these people.

10 Common Fertility Mistakes To Avoid

- **Putting It Off:** Plan early if you want to have kids -- especially if you have a family history of early menopause.
- **Overdoing Intercourse:** Plan to have intercourse every other day or once every three days for optimal results.
- **Over-Exercising:** Over-exercising can be harmful. Instead, do moderate exercise three days a week.
- **Too Much Stress:** Manage your stress by making time for yourself and things you enjoy.
- **Obsessing Over Sex Positions:** No one sex position has been proven to be more effective for conception.
- **Douching:** Douching removes helpful cervical mucus and may even be spermicidal. Stick to soap and water.
- **Living Up Pre-Baby:** Curb your partying before you conceive. Avoid alcohol, cigarettes, fetotoxic medication, and illicit drugs during this time.
- **Waiting Too Long to Get Help:** If you're over 35, seek help after trying unsuccessfully for 6 months. If younger than 35, try for a full year before seeing your doctor.
- **Ignoring Male Health and Lifestyle Issues:** Remember, it takes two to tango.
- **Taking Pregnancy Tests Too Early:** Give your body time before taking a pregnancy test. If you take a pregnancy test too early, you won't get an accurate reading.

Figure 28. How to get pregnant faster

A- HIV-positive women should avoid getting pregnant as much as possible. Therefore, it is recommended that two methods of contraception be used simultaneously in these people (Double method) to minimize the possibility of pregnancy. However, if an HIV-positive woman becomes pregnant, she is prescribed antiviral drugs during pregnancy to try to prevent HIV transmission to her fetus. Of course, prescribing these drugs during pregnancy is associated with risks, while these drugs are very expensive and rare. Antiviral drugs can also be used in babies born to HIV-positive mothers.

B- Health workers are one of the groups at risk of HIV infection. Therefore, guidelines called "standard precautions" have been developed that all health care workers should follow to minimize the risk of HIV transmission.

C- Another high-risk group is injecting drug users who are an important source of HIV infection in the country due to the common use of syringes and needles and other high-risk behaviors. Preventive measures in this group include encouraging addicts to quit, changing injecting drug addiction in less risky ways, and finally distributing free syringes, needles, and condoms among them. These measures are referred to as "harm reduction" strategies.

D- Having sexually transmitted infections such as gonorrhea, syphilis, etc. carries the risk of HIV transmission. On the other hand, treating sexually transmitted infections reduces the risk of HIV infection. Therefore, complete diagnosis and treatment of sexually transmitted infections in patients with them is one of the most important measures to prevent AIDS.

E- People with high-risk behaviors, especially high-risk sexual behaviors, need to be counseled to avoid the risks of HIV infection. Be aware of them and, if necessary, perform diagnostic tests on a voluntary basis. Voluntary counseling and testing is free of charge at Behavioral Disease Counseling Centers across the country.

3- Prevention of HIV infection in the general population, including:

A- Public education about HIV and AIDS and related high-risk behaviors.

B- Ensures the health of blood and blood products.

The most important issue in teaching high-risk behaviors is teaching healthy sexual behaviors.

What are high-risk sexual behaviors?

- Having multiple sexual partners.
- Unusual sexual contact (anal and oral contact).
- Using violence during sexual contact.
- Consumption of alcohol, drugs or psychedelics before sexual intercourse.
- Unprotected sex (not using a condom).

Therefore, in order to prevent HIV and AIDS in society, healthy sexual behaviors should be taught to people, especially adolescents and young people.

Important points in business contacts

1- HIV transmission through healthy skin has not been proven in any place or under any circumstances.

2- No risk of HIV transmission has been observed through close contact with patients, exposure to airborne droplets, and even contact with environmental surfaces.

3- Almost all definite cases of HIV transmission are related to blood or other blood-contaminated fluids, and only two cases were other than this (one case due to pleural fluid and the other due to concentrated culture of HIV).

4- To date, no cases of HBV and HIV transmission through oral respiration have been reported, but to prevent the transmission of herpes simplex and Neisseria meningitis and the theoretical possibility of HIV and HBV transmission in these cases, special masks are used and disinfected after use.

5- Observance of standard precautions in cases of surgery prevents up to 93% of contact with blood.

Occupational contacts that can cause HIV transmission include:

Skin contacts injuries such as needle sinking or cutting with a needle or other sharp object.

1- Contamination of mucous membranes

Infection of unhealthy or damaged skin through scratches or dermatitis (although there are indistinguishable pores in the skin from which HIV can sometimes enter) HIV sources include blood, bloody tissues, tissues and other body fluids such as Semen, vaginal discharge, cerebrospinal fluid, synovial fluid, peritoneal pericardial fluid, and amniotic fluid, all of which can transmit HIV infection to others. In the case of saliva, contact with the saliva of an HIV-infected person is generally not considered a risk factor for HIV transmission if there is no visible blood in it. Contact with tears, sweat and non-bloody stools of an infected person. As a risk factor for HIV transmission, HIV can be transmitted to infants or children through infected human milk. But contact with human milk is not considered an occupational contact for HIV transmission. Studies have shown that the average risk of HIV transmission by needle or other skin damage from sharp objects infected with HIV is about 0.32%. (An infection after 2885 contact through the mucous membrane or damaged skin).

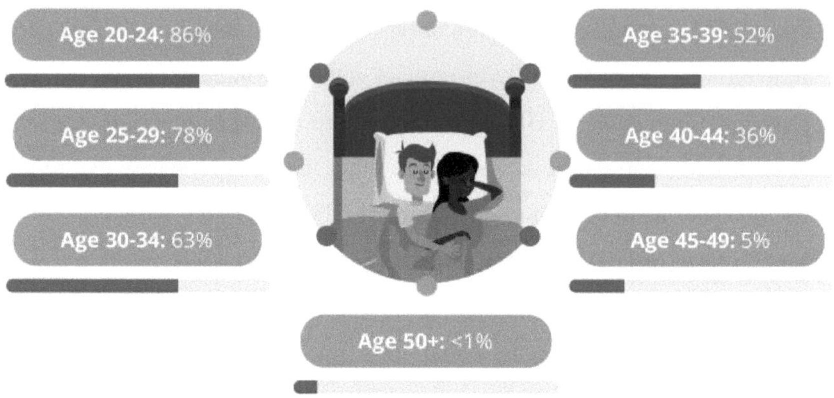

Figure 29. How to Get Pregnant Fast (10 Tips for Faster Conception)

How to prevent the transmission of infection?

As you know, there are two categories of natural flora or bacteria that are naturally present on the skin; The first group of flora or transient and temporary bacteria and the second group with permanent and permanent bacteria. Transient bacteria with normal daily activities are attached to the surface of the skin exposed to the open air and especially under the nails are found in large quantities. Regular hand washing Both pathogenic and non-pathogenic forms of these bacteria are eliminated; But resident bacteria are naturally present in wrinkles with a fixed number and types and are difficult to attach to the skin, and to wash them, you must use brushes and detergents and separate them from the skin. At the same time, temporary bacteria If they remain in large numbers on the skin for a long time, they become resident bacteria; Therefore, regular hand washing is important to prevent the permanent residence of bacteria in the skin. This issue is much more important for medical staff, especially nursing staff who are in constant contact with patients, so it is necessary to pay attention to another issue here. It is the use of jewelry and having long nails that naturally play a special role in the transmission of microorganisms.

Doctors do not touch the ring Recently, in one of the medical centers in Chicago in the United States, a study was conducted on ICU nurses who proved the direct relationship between hand infection and the use of the ring. Jewelry was performed on hand contamination and hygienic detergents were compared, contaminants on the skin of the hand with or without a ring were identified, and the effects of various disinfectants on them were investigated.

The results of this study showed the presence of ring rings on the hand. Nurses increase the accumulation of Staphylococcus aureus, gram-negative bacilli and a variety of Candida (a type of fungus). It is obvious that when the number of rings is more, the amount of contamination will be more. And culture was prepared, interesting results were obtained. These three cleaning agents included wipes soaked in alcohol, dry antibacterial agent and plain soap and water. Any scratches or cuts on the hands, long nails and the use of rings were also mentioned in the report.

While the person is exposed to the roof in subsequent washings, so hand washing with ordinary soap and water is generally recommended for the personal hygiene of hospital staff, and washing with antimicrobial products containing killers or inhibitors of skin organisms only in cases Surgical scrub is also used. This study also showed that contamination of nurses' hands, especially if accompanied by long nails or jewelry, in most cases leads to transmission of the infection to themselves or outside the hospital. According to the latest hygienic washing instructions Hands introduced in October 2003 It is recommended to remove the ring, bracelet and watch before health care and contact with the patient, and their type and sex have no effect on the amount of infection. Transmit it to others and present Reliable statistics on the types of detergents provide the necessary information to attract cooperation, and by conducting experiments and preparing cultivation periodically on the work environment and staff hands to closely monitor and quality control.

Experience shows, the use of Jewelry, especially if accompanied by decorative jewelry, can help transmit microorganisms, can lead to the rupture of sterile gloves and the loss of sterile conditions during work, and increase the possibility of external factors such as blood or secretions and contact with the nurse's skin. ; Of course, there is a problem

here, and that is that many nurses who lose their rings or jewelry while working to prevent contamination may lose them and lose them forever; Therefore, it is wiser to remove them before entering the hospital environment. Although more research is needed to determine the effect of long nails or ornaments on the course of treatment, the Centers for Disease Control (CDC) has specific guidelines. To minimize the possibility of pathogens provided by staff and provided to hospitals;
But as mentioned earlier, the active cooperation of staff based on basic knowledge is more effective than anything else in following the rules. What everyone should know is that although nurses are not directly involved in the practical process of transmitting infection, they can actually be one Complete the chain of transmission of the infection and to prevent this, hand washing should not be underestimated. The issue is much more important than someone saying I do not have time to wash my hands.

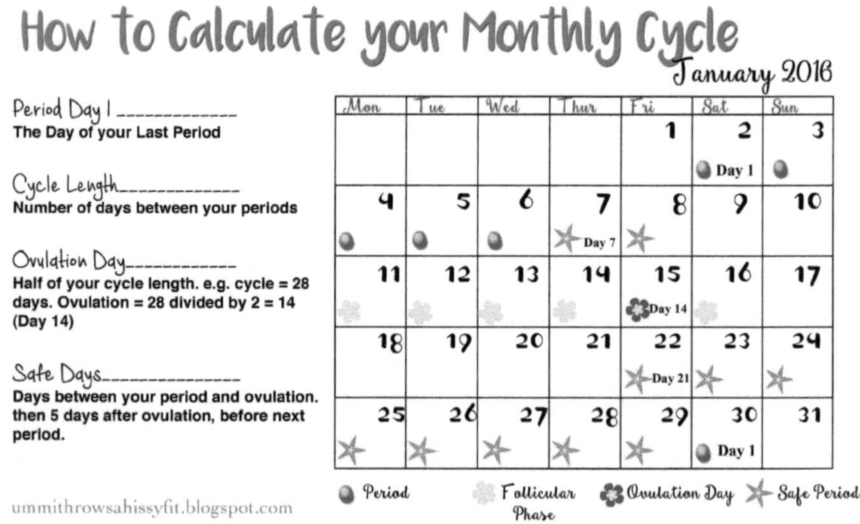

Figure 30. Ummi Throws a Hissy fit: 9 Things to do Before Getting Pregnant

Chapter IV

Telemedicine

Today, information technology has penetrated in all fields and has changed the face of many phenomena. In the field of medicine, the use of this technology is becoming a necessity. Telemedicine is in fact a general concept used to describe various aspects of telemedicine care. The main idea of telemedicine is the transmission of information through electrical signals and the automation of clinical services and consultation. . . By electronic medical equipment. Telemedicine is a new term used to describe the use of electronic information and communication technologies to provide services and support consumers when there is a gap between the client and the service provider. Remote physician goals include improving patient care, improving access and medical care for rural and disadvantaged areas, better access to physicians for counseling, providing facilities for physicians to conduct automated examinations, reducing the cost of medical care, and creating care services. Medicine (geographically and demographically) reduces the transfer of patients to medical centers. Remote ultrasound is a remote pathology, treatment of remote cognitive disorders. Today, telemedicine has advanced to such an extent that it is possible to perform remote surgery. That is, a skilled surgeon in one country, using very strong internet connections and precise technical infrastructure, will be able to perform surgery in one operating room in another country, using robots.

The advent of the Internet and its expansion has made many changes in every science and industry, medical science is no exception to this rule and the Internet, in addition to the effects it has had on its development, has also had significant effects on the development and improvement of medical services. After the advent of the computer and its development, and then advanced information systems such as computer networks and the globalization of the Internet, everyone began to think of using these systems to their advantage. Meanwhile, the medical departments also thought of providing better services to all people through the Internet, because this department was responsible for the most important task. E-health and the provision of health services is one of the fields of science and technology that has a growing growth in the field of health in the world. In fact, e-health is a new term that we need to use a combination of information and electronic communication technology in the field of health and treatment. E-health is a new approach to health care, diagnostics and treatment supported by electronic and communication processes. In this system, all health services are provided, including electronic patient records, telemedicine, evidence-based medicine, informing citizens, informing specialists and virtual medical teams. Telemedicine is a bridge between medical sciences and engineering, in which the medical community uses engineering facilities to promote community health.

Definition

Definitions and terms

The following definition of Telehealth is provided by the United States Office for the Advancement of Telehealth: "Case of health affairs to specialists and patients, public health, implementation and health management."

Telemedicine generally focuses on patient care activities, while Teleheath covers all types of health-related activities. eMedicine has a very close meaning to Telehealth and is actually Telehealth with the difference that it is offered through the Internet. The general concept lies in the fact that all of these activities are the transfer of information on health-related topics that take place between two or more sites through telecommunications technology.

Healthcare Provider: This title refers to people and individuals who provide various services in the field of health and wellness. This collection includes physicians, hospitals, and organizations and institutions providing medical services.

Telehealth components

Telehealth can be divided into three main parts. These three parts also have some overlap with each other. These three are: Informatics, Education, Telemedicine. Now a brief description of each is given.

Telemedicine (which can be said to be easier to set boundaries than others) is telemedicine care through telecommunications technology that includes all aspects of tracking the patient's recovery status remotely through The doctor, prescribing medications and specifying all the activities that the patient should do (such as exercising), questions that the patient wants to ask his doctor and so on.

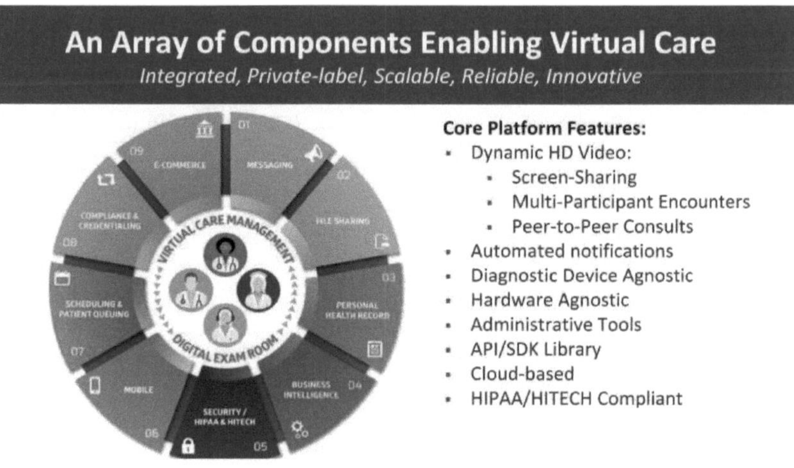

Figure 31. Telehealth Foundations: Applications Across Professions

Education refers to health education that is done remotely. In a division, these trainings can be divided into two parts: trainings that are given to Providers and trainings that are given to patients. In another division, it can be said that these trainings are divided into continuous and continuous trainings or short and cross-sectional trainings, which, if they are for doctors and Provider Healthcare, can be used to teach special courses or specialties. Required (in the form of continuous and continuous training) or for training required in an emergency, outbreak of a disease, or training required by a physician in partial cases (as partial and cross-sectional training) and if for patients They are usually cross-sectional trainings that should be given to them about a particular disease.

Informatics (knowledge and study of methods of processing and sending information) that includes the storage, retrieval and transfer of information to achieve the desired goals, such as databases related to the list of books and ...

The term Tele Medicine was first used in 1920, although its use began about 15 years ago. The British Telemedicine Association defines telemedicine as:

"Providing medical services where distance is an important factor, by professionals using information and communication technology to exchange accurate information in the field of diagnosis, treatment and prevention of diseases and research, taking advantage of the latest achievements in The field of medical services in order to ensure the health of people as much as possible "

Telemedicine is the treatment and treatment of medicine that is applied remotely. Data and information are transmitted through e-mail, post, telephone and fax instead of direct contact. Information transfer can be between patient and physician or between physicians. Telemedicine is a skill that uses multimedia tools and is associated with the use of a large number of modern technologies (live image, live sound, medical data and images, communication systems, texts, photographs and vital parameters). With medicine, it creates a kind of independence of time and place in the field of medical services.

Definition of telemedicine

The use of telecommunication technologies to enhance or accelerate health services is called telemedicine. I operate this system through databases, linking treatment centers and treatment teams or transmitting diagnostic information. In fact, telemedicine uses electronic communications and telecommunications technology to provide and support services such as telemedicine, education and training in health-related fields to specialists and patients, public health development, and health management implementation. Telemedicine is a new term used to describe the use of electronic information and communication technologies to provide services and support consumers when there is a gap between the client and the service provider. It is not really a new concept; it has been around by phone and fax for many years.

This concept has been used since the invention of the telephone before it was used in telemedicine by Thomas Bird in the 1970s. At first, doctors tried to transmit heart and lung sounds to other specialists for telephone examination. This concept includes a range of consultations to more specialized steps such as remote surgery. In this way, it is possible to control and manage crises in the field of health, treatment and health.

When you provide medical advice and diagnoses about a disease to another doctor on the other side of the world and consult with him or her over the Internet, you are actually using telemedicine or when a physician sends you an email. Simply consults a patient on one continent about the illness of one of his patients. In fact, he has used part of this system.

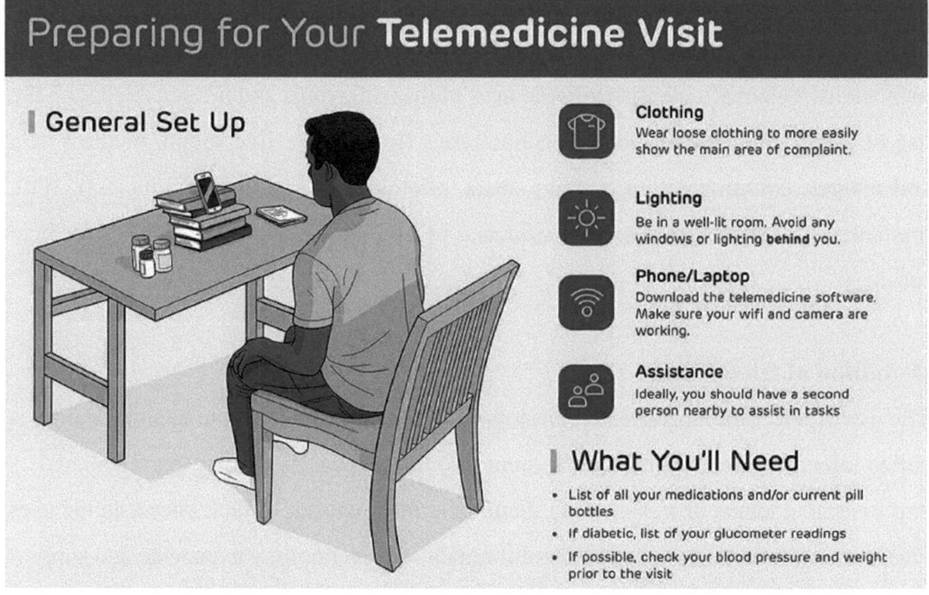

Figure 32. Preparing for Telemedicine Visits: Guidelines and Setup

Communication between physician and patient, remote examination with the help of sending radiological images, sending vital signals and textual and audio reports of the patient's history on the one hand and providing instructions in text or audio or in special cases such as remote surgery as orders Mechanically, the physician forms the cycle of a telemedicine operation. Telemedicine is a skill that utilizes multimedia tools, and medical services can be utilized using a wide range of state-of-the-art technologies, including live video, live sound, medical data and images, communication systems, texts, photographs, and vital medical parameters. Presented from a distance to another place.

Use of medical information through information and communication technology for medical care with the aim of improving the patient's health status. Today there is no clear boundary between the sciences. Many specialties are located between the sciences, including electronic health and telemedicine (telemedicine). In general, this science cannot be considered specific to health sciences or only in the field of information technology. The term telemedicine was first used in 1920. It is used to describe various aspects of telemedicine care. The British Telemedicine Association defines telemedicine as: the provision of health care where Distance is an important factor, used by professionals using information and communication technology to exchange accurate information in the diagnosis, treatment and prevention of diseases and research, taking advantage of the latest achievements in the field of health services in order to provide everything Most people's health.

Telemedicine or telemedicine is a new method in health care, diagnostics and treatment that is supported by electronic and communication processes. The term telemedicine or e-health about fifteen years ago along with terms such as e-mail, e-government.

Telemedicine refers to the use of communication and information technology in medicine with the aim of being able to provide medical services remotely and without the need for routine face-to-face communication between patient and physician. The most important application of telemedicine is also used in electronic counseling, education, preparation of patient databases, artificial intelligence and support for the management of medical systems.

Telemedicine or telemedicine refers to the transmission of information through electrical signals and the automation of clinical services and counseling with the help of electronic medical equipment. In general, telemedicine refers to the use of communication and information technology in medicine with the aim of Medical services can be provided remotely without the need for routine face-to-face communication between the patient and the physician, which requires the transmission of text, images, audio, video and converted electrical signals. The United Nations uses telemedicine to monitor soldiers Peacekeepers use Although soldiers undergo a medical examination before deployment, they are still exposed to indigenous diseases or accidents. Telecommunications infrastructures have been developed in the target areas, and as a result, soldiers can communicate via ENT and laboratory, ultrasound or teleconferencing. The range of services including medicine, medical and dental diagnoses, ECG results will then be expanded to specialize in neurosurgery, orthopedics, skin diseases and other diseases.

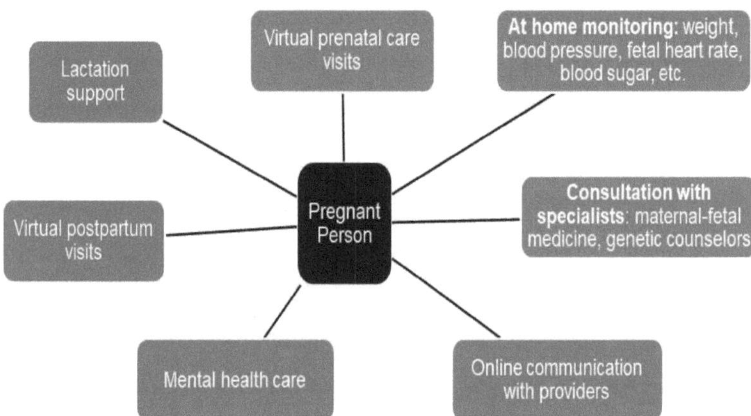

Figure 33. Telemedicine and Pregnancy Care

Types of Telemedicine

Real time (synchronous)

It can be as simple as a phone call to the complexity of robotic surgery. In this type of telemedicine, the two parties need to be present at the same time and establish a real-time communication link between them. One of the most widely used of these is video conferencing equipment. Connected, such as an otoscope that allows the patient to see inside the ear or a stethoscope that allows the patient's heart to hear the sound.

Internal medicine, rehabilitation, cardiology, pediatrics, obstetrics, neurology.

Store-and-forward (asynchronous)

It is taking medical data (such as medical images, vital signals ...) and then sending them to a doctor or specialist for offline examination. Therefore, there is no need for the simultaneous presence of both parties. Specialties in which this type is used: pathology, radiology, dermatology.

History

In 1959, Cecil Whittson launched the first practical telemedicine program. The purpose of this program was to care for the mentally ill and to provide medical education. The idea of telemedicine was proposed to guide the "group therapy" program for the mentally ill. This system was also used to educate medical students. Clinical rooms and classrooms were connected using video tools and a close relationship was provided between the learning environment and the practical conditions of treatment.

In 1968, Massachusetts General Hospital established a microwave video link between the hospital and Boston Logan Airport to give passengers quick access to a doctor if needed. About 1000 patients used this system. In 1978, a satellite network was launched to provide medical coverage in remote parts of Queensland, Australia. Prior to the network, medical consultants used helicopters to reach patients by telephone, radio, or medical services. The main goal of this project was to increase access to medical care in indigenous areas.

The following tools can be used to implement and apply telemedicine on a large scale.

i. Internet network, for education and access to medical information and counseling.
ii. Virtual reality using simulators; In this way, people, with the help of simulation devices, experimentally acquire the necessary skills and training to face real situations and unexpected events; Such as: simulation of medical emergencies on the battlefield or in the event of an earthquake, flood, fire.
iii. Use video conferencing and do video consultations.

iv. The use of Pocket PCs and PDAs by paramedics, doctors and others to send the necessary information and get immediate advice from anywhere in the world.
v. Using smart clothes to send the person's condition to the medical team; Such as sending the status and geographical location of soldiers and war wounded to aid workers.

The history of the use of communication technology in the treatment process dates back to the mid-eighteenth century. At that time, telegraphs and telephones were used to communicate between members of the medical team.

The first organization to seriously address the issue of telemedicine was the US National Aeronautics and Space Administration, NASA. They needed to monitor the health of their astronauts in different situations. The astronauts were connected to centers such as Mir Station with the help of telemedicine systems, and then the station was connected to Earth, and specialists from medical centers on the ground monitored the astronauts' health.

During space travel, scheduled video conferences were usually held privately between astronauts and their physicians, during which physicians examined their physical condition. Some stages of this process require complex hardware subsystems, such as Remote surgery, which in addition to transmitting text, audio and video, requires the conversion, transmission and retrieval of complex and precise mechanical commands. However, parts of telemedicine, such as medical advice, are easy to do. When your doctor consults a colleague on another continent by sending a simple email about your condition, he or she is actually using part of a Telemedicine system.

The main application of telemedicine.

Telemedicine has a wide variety of applications and technologies that have been developed to increase the health and well-being of the individual in society. This phenomenon can be determined by the type of information sent (such as clinical trials and radiographs), how to send this data and the meaning and Find meaning. This phenomenon can be used in practice in the following cases:

• Natural disasters and wars.
• Development of health in difficult areas.
• Control of chronic diseases.
• Air flights.
• Sea voyages in wars.
• Diagnosis, treatment, control, follow-up and consultation.
• Educate service providers and people.
• Medical information resources including a variety of databases and medical databases.

Tele Medicine goals

• Improve patient care.
• Improving access and medical care for rural and disadvantaged areas.
• Better access to doctors for advice.
• Provide facilities for physicians to conduct automated examinations.
• Reducing the costs of medical care, patient transfer and accommodation in a medical center.
• Establishment of medical care services (at the geographical and large population level).
• Reducing the transfer of patients to medical centers.
• Creating a managed care environment in hospitals and treatment centers.

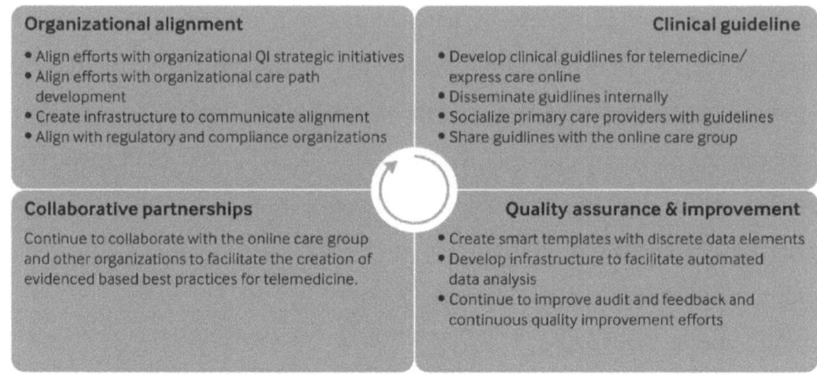

Figure 34. Ensuring Clinical Quality in Telemedicine

History of telemedicine

In 1959, Cecil Whittson launched the first practical telemedicine program. The purpose of this program was to care for the mentally ill and to provide medical education. The idea of telemedicine was proposed to guide the "group therapy" program for the mentally ill. This system was also used to educate medical students. Clinical rooms and classrooms were connected using video tools and a close relationship was provided between the learning environment and the practical conditions of treatment.

In 1968, Massachusetts General Hospital established a microwave video link between the hospital and Boston Logan Airport to give passengers quick access to a doctor if needed. About 1000 patients used this system. In 1978, a satellite network was launched to provide medical coverage in remote parts of Queensland, Australia. Prior to the network, medical consultants used helicopters to reach patients by telephone, radio, or medical services. The main goal of this project was to increase access to medical care in indigenous areas.

The following tools can be used to implement and apply telemedicine on a large scale.

i. Internet network, for education and access to medical information and counseling.

ii. Virtual reality using simulators; In this way, people, with the help of simulation devices, experimentally acquire the necessary skills and training to face real situations and unexpected events; Such as: simulation of medical emergencies on the battlefield or in the event of an earthquake, flood, fire.
iii. Using video conferencing and conducting video consultations.
iv. The use of Pocket PCs and PDAs by paramedics, doctors and others to send the necessary information and get immediate advice from anywhere in the world.
v. Using smart clothes to send the person's condition to the medical team; Such as sending the status and geographical location of soldiers and war wounded to aid workers.

Telemedicine goals and e-health

1- Improve patient care.

2- Improving access and medical care for rural and disadvantaged areas.

3- Better access to doctors for advice.

4- Provide facilities for physicians to conduct automated examinations.

5- Reduce the cost of medical care.

6- Establishment of medical care services (at a large geographical and demographic level).

7- Reducing the transfer of patients to medical centers.

8- Creating a managed care environment in hospitals and medical centers.

9- On the ship, inside the plane.

10- War zones.

11- Far prisons.

Problems and obstacles

• Increase the possibility of misdiagnosis.

• Hardware costs.

• Need a good communication network.

• Staff training: One solution is to include Telehealth training in medical school curricula.

• Educate patients and users: Because many people do not know about TeleHealth and its capabilities and limitations, so the benefits of this system should be taught to them.

Major Barriers to Telemedicine Development.

Despite rapid growth, there are still significant barriers to the normal use of Telemedicine. Here are some of the obstacles:

Formality and legality

In many parts of the world, there is still no legal background to implement and use eMedicine services, and there are still legal issues that do not allow or provide the necessary support to those active in this field. However, it is hoped that this problem will gradually disappear over time.

Required bandwidth

Healthcare requires a lot of data transfer that is very large (such as certain types of photos and videos). This requires a lot of bandwidth (for example, to transfer some type of image to a bandwidth of about 75 (Mb / s) is required). It is clear that many countries in the world are having difficulty in providing such bandwidth. To this end, experts in this field try to solve this problem along with the development of other IT fields.

Development of multilingual systems

Today, most services in this field are limited to a few specific languages in the world and many people around the world are deprived of these services due to unfamiliarity with these languages. For this reason, in order to make these services universal, this problem must be overcome.

Economic efficiency

In many parts of the world, due to the lack of proper IT infrastructure, there are many economic problems to implement and provide eMedicine services, and even the implementation of a project in this area may cause economic losses. For this reason, before implementing any project in this field, it should be considered economically.

Payment for services

There are many problems in this regard. It should be clear where the initial costs of implementing a project come from and how they are repaid. How to charge for services from users of these services. What about the situation of the doctors and the institutions that provide their services in this way, and many other problems that need to be solved with proper planning and the creation of appropriate laws?

Available patterns

Because it does not take long to provide Healthcare services through the Internet, there are still not enough suitable and tested models in this field, and we should try to identify the best ones and implement them in the community over time and implement different models.

Moral barriers

Because the people of the world are of different species and with different beliefs, each of them has its own morals and anti-morals. Because the provision of services over the Internet blurs geographical boundaries, a service or medical activity may not be morally problematic in one area but immoral in another (for example, the issue of abortion in One state is banned and the other is free).

Social status

It should be noted that before providing any service through the Internet, including Healthcare services, prepare the people of the community to accept such service. If this is not done, many problems (economic, social, etc.) will arise. For example, people should be persuaded to share their problem online with their doctor and trust the doctor's prescription instead of going to a doctor's office or a hospital during a minor illness.

Differences and national and legal contradictions in the world

The last problem to be addressed is the important issue of national disputes and conflicts that exist in the field of Healthcare laws. Therefore, a doctor cannot provide the same services all over the world, but in providing these services, he must always pay attention to the country and even the region in question. Of course, this is not a problem in countries that are legally and culturally similar (such as Canada and Australia), but in other places it can cause many problems. Telemedicine users have a huge role to play in speeding up and advancing it, because they take a big risk in using Telemedicine services, and that is trusting such services. Because this issue has a major difference with other issues, and that is that the activities carried out here have a direct impact on patients' lives. Of course, this existing risk causes consumers of these services to try to significantly increase their role in this, and this is not possible except by increasing their information. Therefore, the direction of services is shifted to educational services, and the activities carried out in this sector will increase significantly.

Types of Tele Medicine services

1- Remote consultation.

2- E-learning.

3- Remote monitoring.

4- Remote surgery.

Remote consultation

Telemedicine has the largest share of Tele Medicine due to its simplicity and wide range of applications. All communication facilities, including telephone, fax, e-mail, Internet chat, message page, etc. can be used for remote consultation. Of course, it should be borne in mind that the Internet has no boundaries and as much as possible Get useful information from it, there is wrong and inaccurate information in it. Such information should always be avoided, as well as fake doctors and sites without medical credentials.

E-learning

E-learning is defined as: E-learning is the use of information technology tools in the training and education of human resources. Information technology tools include all computer networks, including the Internet, all types of training CDs, and all software. Physicians, of course, have to leave the field to attend existing classes. The time cost of attending classes, plus the time spent on long-distance or intercity travel to attend classes, can be significantly reduced by using electronic systems. Also, the cost of accommodation and educational space is reduced with the help of e-learning.

Remote monitoring

Sending medical images online or offline, vital patient signals via video conferencing, is one of the main methods of remote monitoring. Types of remote monitoring procedures include: Remote Radiology, Remote Pathology, Remote Cardiology, Remote Home Care, and other systems that are less common, such as remote electrogastrography.

Remote radiology

The concept of digital radiology was introduced by Dr. Paul Capp in the early 1970s. But the lack of the necessary technology prevented the development of digital radiology until the early 1980s. A digital radiology department consists of two parts: The Radiology Information Management System (RIS) and the Digital Images section. Radiological information management is a subset of the Hospital Information Management System (HIS), which includes information about each patient. The digital imaging component, also known as Picture Arching & Communication Systems (PACS), includes image capture, image archiving, image transfer, image reconstruction, image display, and image processing. It is formed in different categories that are connected through the network.

Imaging systems

In the last two decades, we have witnessed the development and growth of various imaging methods such as: ultrasound, MRI, computed radiography (CT), all of which are digital. These computer imaging techniques make up only 30 percent of medical images, and the rest are x-rays. The images obtained from this method are non-digital and in order to be used in PACS system and digital radiology, they must be digitized with the help of digitizers (Laser Scanner, Solid State Camera, Drum Scanner, Video Camera, Photodiode detector, Charged Coupled Device).

Obtaining data

One of the problems with the PACS system is that it receives images and reports them from medical devices. The reason for this is that the manufacturers of imaging devices do not meet the existing standards. To solve this problem, a computer is used which is located in the general block in the Interface section. This computer, which is located between the device and other parts of PACS, isolates the device from the whole system. This computer has three main functions:

- Capture video data from the imaging device.
- Convert received data to standard ACR - NEMA or DICOM format.

• Send standard data to the PACS controller.

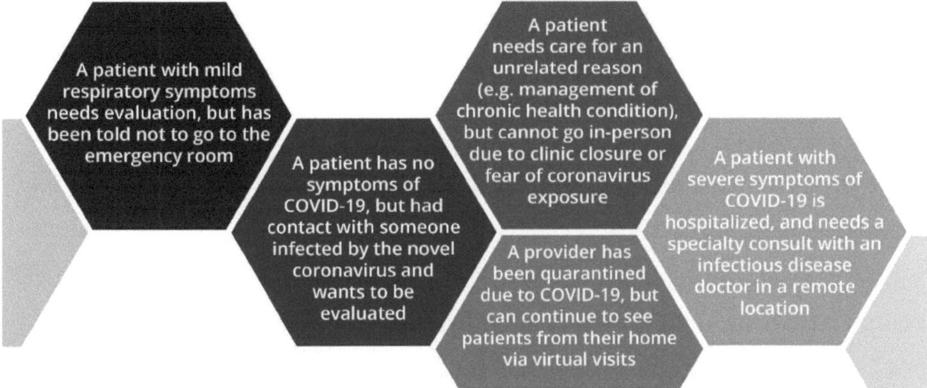

Figure 35. Opportunities and Barriers for Telemedicine in the U.S. During the COVID-19 Emergency

PACS controller

The main components of this section are: database server and archive section. Some functions and functions of the PACS controller:

• Receive images of a medical study taken from a computer.

• Extract text information contained in images.

• Update system network information.

• Determine which display stations the images should be sent to.

• Automatic retrieval of comparative images from the archive.

• Determine the optimal contrast and brightness for displaying images.

• Compress images.

• Archiving new images on optical discs.

• Delete archived images taken from the computer.

• Ability to retrieve images from different workstations.

How to communicate

In general, a computer uses certain standards and protocols to communicate with peripherals or another computer, some of which are:

- IEEE 488.1 / 2 standard
- Serial
- VXI
- SCSI
- LAN

There are also different topologies for connecting computers, such as the bass topology, the ring topology, and the star topology.

Picture Archiving and Communication Systems (PACS), Radiology

PACS, PACS radiology, is a computer-based image storage and retrieval system that can image images from several different diagnostic imaging modalities such as MRI, CR, digital radiography, digital angiography, nuclear medicine, and ultrasound. Save and retrieve images in digital format. PACS includes payment and image display stations connected to image archiving tools and networking capabilities. PACS Possibility of transmitting digital image to any of the hospitalized or out-of-hospital networked wards via WAN or the Internet, physician direct access to stored images and thus reducing physician dependence on technicians; Provides simultaneous access for surgeons, reference physicians, and emergency department personnel to images and centralized advice on comparing multiple methods. Digital image storage can also help with video storage problems such as lost and re-captured videos, the need to copy videos, the large volume of video, and the high cost of video.

In most cases, PACS communicates with the Hospital Information System (HIS) and Radiology Information System (RIS) to communicate images with the patient's demographic information, income and expenditure, and administrative / administrative functions, as well as the tele radiology system for Facilitate the transmission and reception of patient images and information from remote areas. The collaboration of these systems can improve communication between departments and, ultimately, improve the efficiency and quality of patient care in the hospital.

Work Principles

Because most custom systems are tailored to the personal tastes of their users, the appearance of these systems is different. PACS generally consists of host computer communication tools, image archiving tools, and display stations that connect to the communication network. Each network component has a computer or processor that controls image transmission. The speed of transmission depends on the type of computer and the method of networking media that establishes the connection between these components. It will cost $ 5 to $ 20 million. The mini-PACS is typically priced at $ 500,000 to $ 1 million and can be purchased as a wide range of extensible modular systems. Multiple mini-PACSs can then be integrated to form a larger network.

Radiology Information Systems

A radiology information system (RIS) performs the following functions:

- Registration and follow-up of the patient.
- Examination schedule.
- Report the results and prepare a report.
- Movie archive management.
- Database management and conversions.
- Auditing and accounting.
- Automatic faxing of reports to reference physicians.

Some RISs are specific to one method - for example, a mammogram report.

Most systems can be connected to the hospital information system to allow the patient to automatically accept demographic information, transmit examination information, and retrieve patient history. RIS can reduce the time and cost required to process information that was previously done manually. RIS should be able to connect to PACS and tele radiology systems to facilitate clinical diagnosis, image management of patient information, and educational / research applications.

Telemedicine systems - radiology

Tele radiology systems (remote radiology), electronic transmission of radiobiological images and consulting texts, from one place to another. Tele radiology systems are designed to facilitate rapid diagnosis and consultation by imaging specialists and to enable communication between different parts of the hospital and other departments, physicians' homes or clinics through telephone lines, digital networks, and / or transmissions. Microwave or satellite. Because it is possible to transmit image data over thousands of miles, remote hospitals and emergency medical centers that do not have a resident radiologist can transfer the relevant images to a larger hospital for review and interpretation for proper review and interpretation. In this regard, be done. Remote radiology enables two-way online consultation and allows the radiologist to provide services to several independent radiology clinics or mobile centers without leaving the hospital's radiology department. tele radiology is also used by the military in times of war and by emergency medical personnel in the event of natural disasters, thereby improving emergency diagnosis and treatment.

Video conferencing systems, telemedicine

Telemedicine videoconferencing systems are used to diagnose and prescribe medical treatment to patients in remote locations, remote clinical counseling, medical staff training, and office / business affairs. Telemedicine, or telemedicine, can be as simple as a phone call between staff or sending a fax from a cardiologist to a primary care physician, or as complex as a simultaneous video examination by doctors hundreds of miles apart. Today, the most common use of this technology is training and management. Of course, the uses of telemedicine technology are increasing. Nowadays, in cases where images (such as radiographs, pathology slides) and other information about the patient are taken on one side and sent to the memory system on the other side for later review, in radiography, tele pathology and Tele dermatology is

used. Telemedicine systems have also been used in surgical, ophthalmological, dental, cardiological, psychiatric and emergency medical consultations. Patient examinations are conducted using devices such as medical earphones, ophthalmoscopes, and examination cameras connected to the telemedicine system, and at the same time allow the physician at a remote location to access patient examination information and communicate with the physician. Consult an examiner, physician assistant or nurse.
The use of telemedicine videoconferencing technology can reduce the costs of specialist travel and patient transfer and the time required to diagnose the disease and make treatment decisions. The usefulness of telemedicine technology, especially in integrating the clinical resources of health-hospital systems, overcoming geographical barriers and shortage of medical personnel when treating patients in disasters and war situations, and providing health care services to patients in isolated areas (such as rural areas). And prisons) has been proven. Wider adoption and use of telemedicine technology is expected to increase the quality of care and reduce the cost of international specialist care.

Patient Identification and Security Systems

Patient safety equipment warns personnel in cases where an infant is taken out of the infant room or the disease is lost. These devices are designed for use in all types of health care centers, including hospitals, nursing homes for the elderly and disabled, and long-term care centers and relief centers. Patient monitoring provides more freedom of action for them as well as health care personnel and allows patients to feel more independent. Getting lost and fleeing is one of the costliest hazards that long-term care centers face. Risks that threaten the health of people in any situation where patients or residents of these centers are able to move without assistance, as well as in cases of long-term disorders. Risks to the health of people in any situation where patients or residents of these centers are able to move without assistance, as well as in cases of cognitive impairment, such as dementia, stroke, drug or alcohol disorders or mental illness.

Fugitives are identified with missing persons through aimless, overt, and often repeated attempts to leave the building and its grounds. People prone to getting lost should be identified quickly. Patients in rehabilitation centers and nursing home residents with cognitive impairments may wander the stairs or insecure areas, leave the building to find their home or familiar surroundings, or wander into other occupants' rooms. Situational cognition and confusion may initially occur in new environments. Other causes of confusion include side effects from medications, confusion, stress, noise, loneliness, being in a crowd or unfamiliar environment, or hallucinations. In addition to insurance costs and potential litigation, accidents involving fugitives may draw intense media attention and severely damage the reputation of the health care facility. Neonatal wards, deliveries, neonatal intensive care units (ICUs) or nurseries are evacuated, notifying relevant staff. These devices can also be programmed to alert if they approach an elevator, staircase, or exit to a building, and to locate the labeled child with the push of a button. All measures to prevent infant and child abduction must be taken. In addition to maternity and neonatal classes, it also covers child-related classes, the neonatal or pediatric ICU, and all nursery-related areas. Health care personnel should identify all uncontrolled areas and areas that are not well monitored.

Computerized Provider Order-Entry Systems

The CPOE system is a networked system that allows users to electronically enter the scope of all commands found in paper-based environments, including prescriptions. These systems also provide online decision support and safety alerts online. Authorized users can access clinical information from multiple sources from a single workstation or remote location. This information includes patient-specific diagnostic instructions, such as laboratory and radiological tests; Medication instructions that users can record continuously; Nursing instructions and special instructions. Information can be accessed from workstations within a center, such as a doctor's office or home.

Remote pathology

In this system, it is enough to install a video camera on a laboratory microscope. Because color information is important in pathology and there is no such thing as a radiology film for scanning, methods of scanning images in remote radiology are not applicable here. By installing the camera, any specialist can, when necessary, send the desired slide or slide image on the monitor of the desired centers. Digital video microscopes can also be used to image pathology. The method of capturing an image is exactly the same as capturing an image with a digital camera. In Iran, Behin Research Company has also made such microscopes.

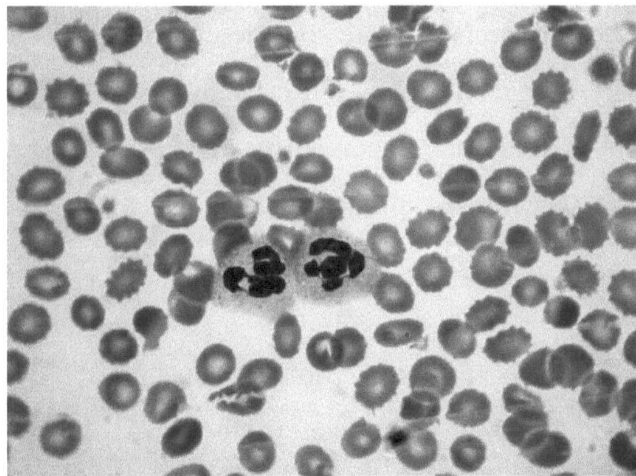

Figure 36. Image obtained from a digital video microscope

Remote cardiology

In the 1970s, the first coupling pacemakers were introduced, which required telemetry to monitor how they worked. Today, patients have small devices with them to send cardiac signals to medical centers.

Basis of telemetry system

The telemetry system transmits information in three stages:

• Signal generation (electrical or otherwise).

• Convert information to the appropriate form.

• data transfer.

A type of telemetry classification is based on the transmitter. Many systems fall into the following three categories:

• Mechanical

• Electric

• Radio

Radio telemetry has an advantage over the other two methods due to the lack of distance restrictions

For a biometric system, two main parts are considered: a transmitter and a receiver. For example, sound energy is transmitted by a microphone and received by a speaker, or light is transmitted by a lamp and received by a photocell, or magnetic fields are transmitted and received by wire couplings.

Modulation systems

Modulation systems in radio telemetry Biomedical signals require the use of two modulators. This means that a lower frequency subcarrier must be present in addition to the VHF, which must eventually transmit the signal from the transmitter. The basis of the two modulators is to create more freedom of action in transmitting and receiving low-frequency biological signals. Sub modulator can be from an FM system or a PWM system. While the ultimate modulator is always an FM system.

Sender

The ECG signal is picked up and amplified by three flexible electrodes attached to the patient's chest and used to modulate the frequency of a 1 KHz sub carrier. The resulting signal is emitted by one of the electrode leads (RL), which acts like an antenna. The transmitter input circuit is protected against large amplified pulses that may result from defibrillation.

ECG input amplifier

The ECG input amplifier acts as an ac couple for the next steps. The coupling capacitor not only limits the dc voltage but also the cut-off frequency of the system, which is usually 0.4 Hz.

Receiver

The receiver consists of an RF amplifier, an RF filter and an image frequency remover.

Multi-channel telemetry system

Solving medical measurement problems often requires the simultaneous transfer of several parameters. A multi-channel telemetry system is used for this application.
In this method, we are allowed to transfer parameters simultaneously, which depends on the number of channels required. ECG, heart rate, respiration rate, temperature and blood pressure are among these parameters. In multi-channel telemetry, the number of sub carriers used is equal to the number of signals received, so each channel has its own modulator. The RF unit, which is the same for all channels, converts different frequencies into transmission frequency bands. Similarly, the receiver unit includes an RF unit and a demodulator for each channel. PWM is more suitable for multi-channel biometer systems. Some systems are not sensitive to the frequency shifts of carrier waves and have high noise immunity. FM systems, although they may have low power consumption and high linear stability, are very complex and expensive. The separator technique usually requires complex and expensive filters.

Bluetooth technology

Bluetooth, which some have translated into Persian as blue tooth. It is a standard for radio waves used for wireless communication of mobile and fixed electronic devices. The Bluetooth transmitter operates in the ISM (Industrial, Scientific, Medical) frequency band at 2.4 GHz binary FM modulation. Data is transmitted in both simple and augmented at speeds of 1 and 2-3 Mbps, respectively. In this system, a radio channel is divided between a group of Bluetooth-enabled devices. It is a master device that synchronizes everyone with its clock and frequency, and the rest are slaves. This network is a Piconet with a Master and a few Slaves. If we connect several Piconets, we have a Scatternet. One of the ways that Bluetooth-enabled devices use to prevent interference with other devices is to send very weak signals as small as one milliwatt, while powerful cell phones have the ability to send signals as large as 3 watts. This feature limits the Bluetooth communication range to about 10 meters.

- is a standard for radio waves? The Bluetooth transmitter operates in the ISM frequency band (Industrial, Scientific, Medical) at 2.4 GHz binary FM modulation.
- Two simple and augmented, transmission at speeds of 1 and 2-3 Mbps, respectively.
- is a reference device (Master) and the rest and slave.
- Master A Master and a few Piconet Slave.
- Multiple Piconet Scatternet.
- Range 10 meters.
- Obstacles must be non-metallic.
- Interference does not stop communication.
- Cardiology telephoto with Bluetooth.

But what does this really have to do with blue teeth?

Harald Bluetooth was King of Denmark in the late 10th century. He united Denmark and part of Norway and recognized Christianity in Denmark. The choice of a name for a standard indicates what major Scandinavian and Baltic companies have played a role in the communications industry. This naming was done with the aim of uniting the communication and computer industry.

The patient is collected at the ECG Cardiology Center. ECG signals are then transmitted to a modem over a short distance (10-20 m) by Bluetooth technology. From there it is sent to a web server.

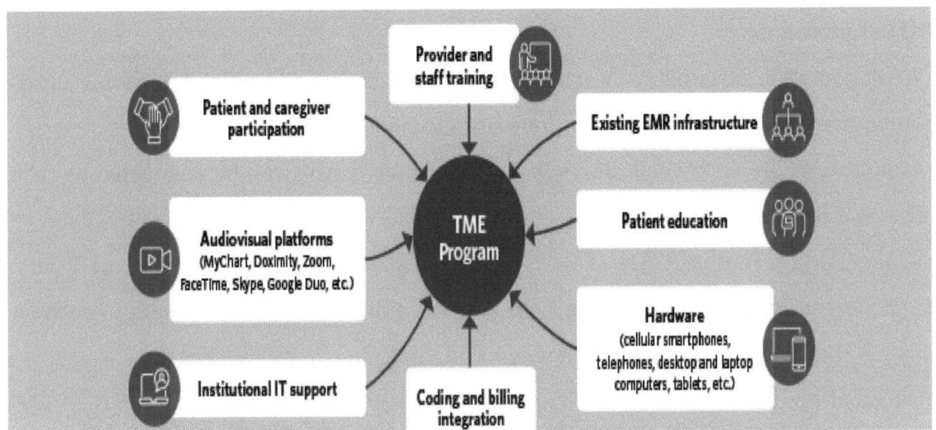

Figure 37. New toolkit provides rapid implementation guide for adopting telemedicine during COVID-19

ISDN (Integrated Services Digital Network) lines

Digital services that can support video, data, and audio at the same time are called ISDNs. ISDN standards are defined by the International Telecommunication Union (ITU). ISDN lines are actually regular telephone lines. There are two types of ISDNs. There are two types of ISDN:

- BRI (Basic Rate Interface).
- PRI (Primary Rate Interface).

BRI

A BRI line uses two type B channels and one type D channel. Each B channel has a speed of 64 Kbps and these channels are used to send and receive data and audio. The type D channel has a speed of 16 kbps and is used to communicate the signal. Therefore, the maximum velocity of a BRI is 2B + D

$2B + D = 2 \times 64 + 16 = 144$ Kbps

Of course, this type of line is mostly known with the same 2B speed of 128 kbps, because a combination of two B channels provides a speed of 128 Kbps.

BRI applications

• With complete installation of appropriate hardware and software, a desirable video conferencing can be performed for long distances with it.

• Connecting LANs to each other: With these lines, LANs can be connected to each other and form a WAN.

• Connecting a remote LAN: This is also one of the interesting features of ISDN. Suppose you have a LAN that is a long way from the server and you want to connect that LAN to your server. One good way to do this is to use ISDN lines.

• Medical application: It usually happens that hospitals transfer radiographs of one patient to another hospital for further information or examination. This takes about 21 minutes with regular modems, while with BRI it takes about 3 minutes.

• Radio and TV applications: With ISDN services, radio stations can report sports news and events from remote stations. Easy installation and adjustment along with reasonable price, these lines have been proposed as a suitable replacement for leased lines.

PRI

The PRI line has 23 type B channels (64 Kbps) and one D channel with 64 Kbps speed, which is a total of 1,544 Kbps of total line bandwidth. In the United States, this line is used instead of the T1 line (although in Europe, the number of B channels is 30 and the total speed is 2.048 Mbps).

PRI applications

• Connect two central switches (such as PBX) to each other.

• Create video conferencing with good audio and video quality.

• Connect LANs and form a WAN

Benefits of ISDN

• More transfer speeds.

• Less noise due to digital.

• Less communication time (2 to 4 seconds).

• Use the Caller ID service (for showing the caller number), for telephone services.

Because ISDN is a digital service, the distance from the user to the center should not be more than 5.5 km.

Sending heart signal via telephone line

This project has been done in the framework of the final project of Jalil Mazlum Master's degree at Amirkabir University of Technology.

The prototype built for the project includes a small board that can take 12 standard ECG signal derivatives and has connections to electrodes. In addition to receiving the signal, the board performs processes such as filtering, digitizing and amplifying, and finally sends this information over the phone.

This device has several operating modes. In the first case, the device starts dialing as soon as it connects to the telephone line. Dialing is done intelligently and all the steps that a person follows in dialing are performed. Finally, as soon as the connection is made, a two-way communication is established between the device and the receiving station. The receiving station is actually a computer that stores or displays information using software designed by the device manufacturer. A series of hand shaking signals are exchanged between the sender and the receiving computer. Then the signal capture and transmission begin online. In another mode, the device picks up the signal and stores it in its memory and then sends it when needed. Information is collected from each derivative for 13 seconds, but only about 6 seconds during transmission. In another mode, the same device connects directly to the computer without a telephone line (any computer on which the software is installed can work with the system via a serial port). The receiver only needs one computer device.

This device has been tested in Imam Khomeini Hospital under the supervision of 5 experienced cardiologists and has had 300 hours of successful clinical activity, and the specialists have confirmed the steps of receiving and sending the signal and keeping the signal unchanged in the transmission process.

Transmission of heartbeat signal via mobile phone.

A team of researchers from the University of Illinois at Urbana-Champaign and Lucent Technologies has developed a way to extract data about the human breath and heart from cellular signals. In this way, these signals can be monitored through the telephone line. Their idea is to use the mobile phone as a miniature radar that uses the Doppler phenomenon. They can monitor the movement of the chest and how it moves from the frequency shift generated by the received signal. From this information you can get information about both how you breathe and your heart rate.

Remote home care

Most people with cardiovascular disease and chronic respiratory disorders need such care. The initial design of the telemedicine system includes the patient's home as a central station, a station for the participating medical caregivers, and a communications service provider.

The minimum equipment required includes a device for entering information (such as blood pressure) and a communication device for exiting information (telephone line). In more advanced cases, there are devices to monitor the patient's vital factors, an image system for counseling, and an ISDN telephone line for simultaneous transmission of information and images.

Wireless device for accessing medical information.

This section describes the Bluemedica system, which provides physicians and nurses with mobile access and information collection in the hospital. They get the latest patient information from anywhere in the hospital. Bluemedica is always able to determine the information stored in HIS. Part of Bluemedica is a wristband that measures and collects patient health information and provides a list of examinations and treatment admissions.

The first goal is to design a local area network for mobility and public access to information stored in the information system. Bluetooth technology has been used to achieve this goal. The benefits of Bluetooth technology include: low power consumption, low electromagnetic radiation and easy understanding.

Telemedicine and Telehealth Facts

1 One in 10 Americans uses telemedicine.

2 Patients 18 to 24 use telemedicine more than any other age group.

3 Only 5.3 percent of seniors use telemedicine.

4 Telemedicine is less popular in rural areas.

5 Young women are most likely to use telemedicine.

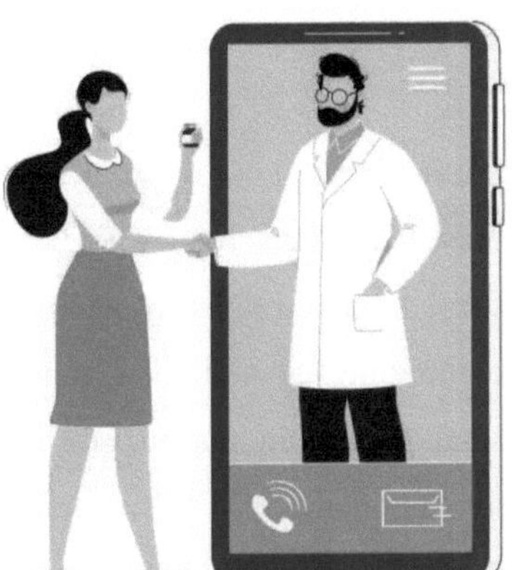

Figure 38. Telemedicine

Health smart card history

Since the mid-1980s, about one hundred pilot projects using smart cards for medical purposes have been implemented, mainly in Europe, South America, Japan and Australia. The information of these cards was divided into two groups of managerial information and medical information. In most of the initial plans, a specific group of patients or certain diseases were covered in Belgium for HEMA CARD. For example, in France for DIALYBRE CARD patients, blood patients in Germany for dialysis patients use DIAB CARD. The number of countries that have a health card-based e-health system is not large; In addition, the scope of use of the card in these countries includes a wide range from a small health care complex to a state and even a country.

Medical records, medical records, insurance records, possibility of paying expenses, possibility of paying insurance premiums and the like are also different.

What is a smart card?

Simply put, a smart card is a small, non-manipulative computer; This little computer has a chip. The chip includes a central processing unit and some amount of permanent memory, some of which, on most cards, is unmanageable (or sometimes hidden), and the rest for applications that can communicate with the card is available.

Health smart card

It is the keyboard and screen. The electricity needed to start this personal computer is provided by the card reader system when the card is connected to it. The card reader system communicates with this computer through the inputs installed on the card. Like any personal computer, smart cards have an operating system that is stored inside the card when it is made, and this operating system is usually not changeable (although other data on the card will be changed or added later). The smart card, because it is a complete computer, can perform encryption operations within itself. One of the most important "security" features of these features is the smart card features.

What is an IBBC barcode chip?

An advanced barcode chip recently developed by a research team (consisting of several different laboratories) has revolutionized medical diagnostic testing. In less than ten minutes, with the help of a drop of blood, the chip can determine the concentration of proteins, such as proteins that appear in the blood due to heart disease or cancer and are a hallmark of these diseases.

IBBC1 This device, as it is known, is made by members of the Cancer Bio Nano systems Center 2, one of the top eight Nano cancer technology centers the size of a slide. IBBC 3 (CCNEs) is microscopic and made of glass. With 1 IBBC (Integrated Blood-Barcode Chip) 2 Nano - systems Biology Cancer Center 3 Nano Technology Cancer Center is silicon.

The surface of this chip is designed in such a way that the flow of micro fluid can move in it. After a drop of blood enters the system through this microscopic canal, the protein-rich plasma is separated and protein biomarkers are measured. Using this chip speeds up measurements and reduces their cost.

How can using this chip reduce costs?

In conventional tests, one or more blood vials are taken from the patient, centrifuged in the laboratory, and divided into cell and plasma sections, then the plasma section is used to perform protein assays, which is a difficult and laborious task; So that if it is done in a hurry, it will take several hours.

Each diagnostic kit costs $ 50 for a protein. With the help of IBBC chip, while reducing time and cost, it is possible to measure the blood of eight people at the same time, and in each measurement, many proteins are also measured. As blood enters the ABC and enters the microscopic canal, its plasma is directed to narrow canals that branch off from the main canal. They do plasma well. The plasma then passes through barcodes that contain a series of lines 20 microns wide. Here, the barcodes make it possible to separate a specific protein from the plasma. The volume of the protein will be determined by the concentration of the protein.

Applications of this chip to date

Researchers have used this technology to measure HCG, which increases up to 100,000 times during pregnancy. It has also been used to measure protein biomarkers in patients with prostate and breast cancer. These biomarkers are different in different patients; For example, a woman with breast cancer will have different biomarkers with a man with prostate cancer, and a woman with benign breast cancer will have different biomarkers with a woman with malignant breast cancer. Allows physicians to administer specific treatments to their patients and to understand patients' responses to medications. The IBC is currently used in patients with glioblastoma (an advanced type of brain tumor). The information on this barcode chip is read using a scanner and is also used in gene and protein expression research.

The role of the IBC in the laboratory system

Automated and mechanized health system

Electronics: The general design idea of this device is based on ATM systems in which the IBC chip (ATM) of banks is embedded. So that health users only enter the mechanized health system by referring to the headquarters of these devices and placing their health card in the relevant entrance, and then by selecting the desired test option or a general check of a drop of their blood in the relevant position. The test is performed in less than ten minutes and the response is recorded online in the person's electronic file, and then based on the test results, the person automatically receives the necessary warnings or medical advice. For example, if a person has high blood sugar, he / she will be informed about it and the system will provide the person with the complications of this disease and the necessary strategies and recommendations for its improvement. At present, a person only has to spend time traditionally performing simple cycles of blood factor tests and enduring the pain of a medical diagnosis laboratory.

How to use this chip in an automated laboratory device?

This chip is connected to the scanner system with a simple connection and has the ability to be replaced automatically, so that after every 8 visits, the chip is replaced automatically. The system installed on this system is as follows: After inserting the card and selecting the desired option, the door of the chip station is opened and then closed by loading the input and the necessary pressure to push the blood cells into the barcodes is applied automatically. After the results are read by the scanner, the data analysis enters the electronic health system online and is stored in the individual's medical history. Then the person becomes aware of his health and can study the side effects and effects of drugs on his body. In the meantime, by implementing a kind of written program in the system, the complications of diagnostic factors can be enumerated and prevention strategies can be provided to the patient at the individual level.

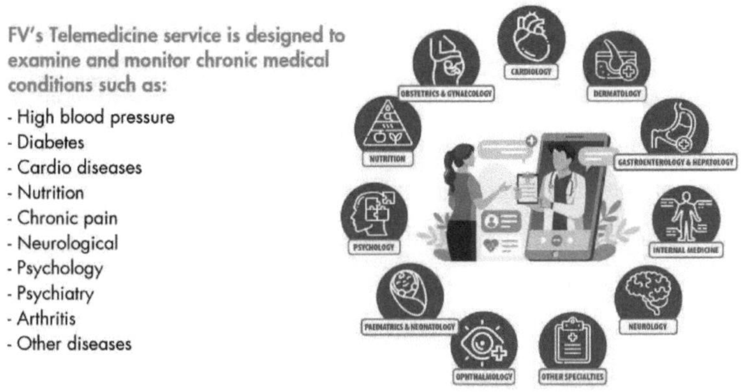

Figure 39. Telemedicine - FV Hospital

The necessity of using the automated laboratory system in rural areas and covering the e-health plan of villages

Usually in rural areas, the level of health is lower and the visit to the doctor is done only in cases of disease. However, in some villages, access to doctors and laboratories is not possible in time, and in addition, the disease has imposed its destructive and irreparable effects on the body. Public Relations and International Affairs of Iran Telecommunication Company.

Health smart card

He informed the offices of communication and information technology services in 10,000 villages of the country. Meanwhile, by installing an automated laboratory device and training the rural population to perform periodic tests at regular intervals, the health level of villages has increased significantly and also the necessary ground for geographical health control and explaining the necessary strategies for prevention in exchange for treatment will be provided.

Establishment of national periodic medical examination plan and health geography map

The National Courses Experimental Plan is a window into the lofty goals of e-health in the statistical community. With the establishment of this plan, the e-government will have a more accurate idea of the medical and pharmaceutical needs and will use more complete strategies to meet them and increase the average life expectancy in the population. In addition, in each geographical area, according to climatic and agricultural conditions and possible nutrition, the amount of blood factors is affected and each area is conducive to a specific type of disease. By creating a health geography map, the possibility of controlling the country's health has increased significantly and researchers' access to this information has become easier. In addition, by repeating the periodic experiments at certain intervals, the effects of the measures taken in this field will appear in the health geography map.

With the creation of a national health site, a database will be provided to provide electronic health information available to users in the electronic field. So that a user by logging in to the national health site and entering his MITWAND health card code will check his medical records consistently and focus more on his personal health. In addition, e-health users by entering this site can be informed of research in the field of medicine and health and improve the level of personal knowledge of the community. In this site, each user, according to his medical history, receives his own warnings and medical advice on his site, and Mitvand corresponds with the recommended doctors on the site at the same time.

Practical examples of telemedicine

Here are some simple examples of telemedicine systems used in practice:

Telemedicine for the treatment of skin diseases (Teledermatology): Diagnosis of skin diseases is made by reviewing the medical history, examination and biopsy. In telemedicine for the treatment of skin diseases, high-resolution color images should be obtained from the site of the complication. The biopsy can be sent by mail to a specialist center. Also, in the case of this type of disease, real-time interaction between specialist and patient is not necessary. At a Teledermatology Center, users are asked to take pictures of their skin condition with a 608 x 832-pixel digital camera and 24 color bits. The examination is performed by 4 dermatologists. In a statistical study of 308 people, 104 of whom also had biopsies, submitted medical records and sent up to 5 images, the average examination time by each physician was 22.6 seconds.

Tele-ultrasound imaging

Ultrasound imaging is a safe, painless, and radiation-free method that has relatively low hardware cost. The operator can easily learn how to take pictures with ultrasound equipment, but he is not able to interpret the resulting images, and this must be done by a specialist. In local clinics, ultrasound imaging of the target areas is performed and the images are viewed in real time by a specialist physician.

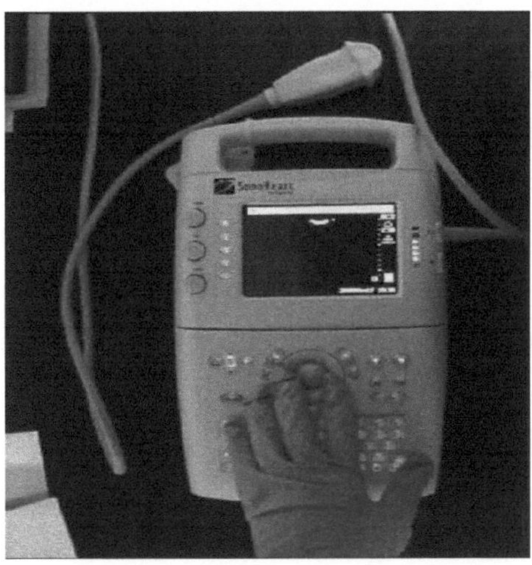

Figure 40. Portable ultrasound device

Telepathology

Pathologists provide slides for information from other relevant specialists. In some cases, such as biopsies of certain parts of the body, it is necessary for experts to exchange opinions quickly and come to an agreement in the shortest possible time. The telemedicine system is used to exchange slide images between pathologists. Digital cameras are attached to microscopes and high quality images are produced from slides. These images are sent to another specialized center. Of course, other clinical details about the patient can be sent with them to other specialists.

Due to the fact that it is difficult for experienced specialists to be present in the above-mentioned places, it is necessary to use a method to benefit from the experience and knowledge of specialists in these places. On the other hand, in many cases, people usually go to the doctor a few days or weeks after the onset of symptoms due to busyness or other causes, as a result, the disease may become more advanced and more difficult to treat. Therefore, if medical services are provided more easily to people, it can be effective in avoiding this problem. Given these points, telemedicine can make a significant contribution to the promotion of public health. Of course, it should be noted that equipment related to the telemedicine system is expensive and in some cases its use is not cost effective. Of course, further advances in technology will make access to telemedicine facilities cheaper and more common. Slowly, in fact, has used part of a telemedicine system. The growing demand for sophisticated and minimally invasive surgeries has created a new branch of research into the use of computer-based information technology as a bridge between the tools used by surgeons and operating devices. The use of computers with advanced surgical aids has fundamentally changed the surgical process in 21st century operating rooms. Integrated Computer Surgery Systems (CIS) allow surgeries to be performed more accurately and with less damage than surgeries. Provides routine and at the same time intelligently and logically tracks and records all relevant information about the patient's condition.

This information, together with the logical follow-up of the patient's output, makes it possible to quantitatively estimate the patient's output and the progress of treatment. This quantity can be considered similar to "total quality management" in manufacturing. The main emphasis on using a surgeon-assisted robot in surgery is to increase the surgeon's capabilities and surgical efficiency. Such systems, which actually operate as a master sleeve and under the command and control of the surgeon, are now referred to as surge traps or surgery by being placed in the surgical console and using the robot commanding tool and looking at the virtual environment of the operation process. It commands the surgery to the robot and the robot performs these operations on the patient's body and in the real environment with features such as accuracy, lack of vibration and fatigue.

Remote surgery

The method is to perform medical surgeries without direct contact of the doctor with the patient during the operation, which is done by giving control to robotic design tools to physicians. The physician can perform the operation at almost any distance while the patient is operated on by robotic surgical instruments with remote control. What enables the physician to control surgery is a strong Internet link that is used to communicate between physicians and surgical instruments, monitors, as well as experienced physicians. The patient undergoing surgery is not left alone with robotic devices, but a physician's assistant is present at the site to observe problems that the physician may not receive due to minor delays in Internet delivery.

Advantages of remote surgery

Remote surgery is performed with the help of a computer, so according to this issue, the strengths of the computer can be combined with human experiences. In a particular surgery, the robotic arm can reduce the effect of natural vibration on the surgeon's hand and increase the surgeon's agility. It is also possible to analyze the inputs applied by the surgeon with a computer and after refining the instructions, apply them to the robotic arm. With the help of a microscope and a computer, the surgeon's range of motion can be reduced to smaller-scale movements, and as a result, more delicate tasks that would not normally be possible for a human agent to perform can be performed using tiny robotic arms. In this case, the patient's body is less damaged during surgery and his recovery occurs faster.

History of remote surgery

The first aid to climbers through telemedicine was in 1996. And then equipping them in 1998. It was performed with instruments that measured the body temperature, pulse and oxygen level of climbers' blood (back-bio). Since then, extensive developments in the application of telemedicine have begun around the world; From simple medical consultations by phone and email to sending radiographs, MRI, CT scans, laboratory results and even remote surgery. In 1988, through small incisions made A small camera was inserted into the body and a small invasive surgery was performed. In 1996, computer robotic surgery was performed. In 2000, the FDA approved the use of a robotic system in the operating room.

In 2001, a doctor in New York operated on the gallbladder of a 68-year-old patient in Strasbourg, France. This was done by remotely guiding a robotic arm. The patient's recovery period was only 2 days, while in open gallbladder surgery the recovery period lasted more than 6 days. The surgery involved two medical teams (in New York and Strasbourg) that were connected by video and high-speed fiber optic line. The two teams were 7,700 miles apart. The time delay of the images received from both sides was displayed on the monitor screen and its amount was less than 200 milliseconds.

The first transatlantic distance surgery in the world.

On September 7, 2001, robot surgery was first performed on a 68-year-old woman. In this surgery, there was a 4,000-mile (7,000-kilometer) distance between the New York surgical team and the hospital at CIVIL Hospital in eastern France, which was traversed by a high-speed fiber-optic line. This operation was performed using the Zeus laparoscopic robotic surgical system and the gallbladder of this woman was removed. The operation lasted only 54 minutes and the 68-year-old woman did not leave for two days after the operation and resumed her normal activities after a week. The robot used in this surgery was designed to perform the operation with the least possible aggression. The surgeon used a Joy stick to control the robots' arm and perform the operation, using images taken by a camera and viewed by a surgeon. The acceptable delay for transmitting image encoding data in such an operation is msec 330, which in the system in question using ATM and RAD'S ACE-2002 technology and NTV (Network Termination Unit) was able to reduce the delay to 115 milliseconds.

This method not only induces a real sense of surgery in the surgeon, but also allows the surgeon to act according to his usual methods and procedures. The surgeon does not need to learn anything new. The hand movements are fast and accurate. The visible movement of the surgical equipment and the force feedback that enters the equipment from the tissue is transmitted to the surgeon exactly by scaling, making microsurgery easier even when the surgeon is with the patient. The system uses color cameras to record stereo images and recordings of surgical sites. And the surgeon at a distance sees these images through special glasses, and the surgeon picks up a pair of remotely controlled manipulators capable of reflecting force, which are connected at the end of the path to a pair of control effectors at the surgical site. The image, sound and force transmitted from the end-effectors to the surgeon induces a sense of presence in him. The surgeon's manipulator consists of two parts. The first part is the general moving part that is outside the body. This part is responsible for the movement of the robot, the second part is the controlled robot. The second part of the slaves is the robot that enters the patient's body. Consequently, it must be very small and at the same time capable of a wide range of motion and relatively large forces. To meet these needs, a wrist 2 degrees of freedom is used that has the ability to rotate around its own axis and move in other directions.

Application of remote surgery in heart surgery

Telemedicine surgery is the result of the adaptation of several technologies such as the Internet, optical fibers and signal transmission.

Open Surgery method

In this method, the chest is split and the surgery is performed directly on the patient's heart. One of the disadvantages of this method is that it may cause clogging of the arteries of the heart and not get enough oxygen to the heart and cause major problems.

Endoscopic Surgery

In this procedure, long, narrow instruments are inserted into the body through small holes and send an image that the surgeon sees on a two-dimensional screen. One of the disadvantages of this method is that the designer has to look at the screen all the time and perform surgery, and this puts a lot of pressure on the surgeon, and the other is that the height of the instruments reduces accuracy and even slight vibration and heart rate of the surgeon amplified. Moves to the end. So after 10-15 years of investing billions of dollars, this method could only make room for low-cost surgeries (such as gallbladder capping, which is a standard procedure) and not for precise surgeries such as heart surgery.

Robotic method

The idea of using robots to help a surgeon is not new. In 1988, minimally invasive surgery (MIS) was performed using small cameras inserted through small holes. On July 11, 2000, the FDA approved the use of the first robotic system, the da Vinci surgical system, in operating rooms. Since then, other robotic systems such as Zeus and AESOP have been developed.

The instruments are inserted into the chest through a small gap (0.5-1 cm) between the ribs. They are inserted into the chest, two of which are the hands of the surgeon, and one of which is the camera that transmits the images to the external unit. It is sent to the other end of the instrument and there, according to the transmitted signal, fine movements are reconstructed and the difference with the endoscope method is that the movement is not produced from the toolbar, but the movement is produced at the tip of the instrument which is about 6-8 mm. There is no mechanical motion transmission at all, but a digital signal is transmitted through the system. The external unit is like a unit on which the surgeon sits and holds the pliers through which the movement of the surgeon's hand is transferred to the indoor unit. Throughout the surgery, he observes the patient through the camera and the pedals that Built-in at the bottom of the unit allows you to adjust the image (zoom in or out, zoom in or out of 3D and change the viewing angle).

It has a pedal device called a clutch, which allows the surgeon to stop the movement and then bring his hand to the desired position. If this is not the clutch, this amount of movement means very strong movement of the instrument inside the body. Even natural vibrations of the surgeon's hand are filtered. The device has a scale for movement that reduces the amount of movement to 1.8, for example, if the movement of the surgeon's hand is 18 cm, the amount of movement of the device will be 10 cm and the dimensions of the image The surgeon sees that it is about 15 times the actual value, and all this increases the accuracy. This surgery can be performed outside the operating room or outside the hospital or even in another city. With this method, specialists in one corner of the world can be used for disease surgery in another place, which is unprecedented in the history of medicine. Of course, there are limitations to remote surgery, such as the interference of sent signals, but the line with signals used by people who are downloading a file or song. There are also problems sending pictures to doctors.

Advantages of Robotic method

• Reduces the long recovery period after standard surgery. As a result, postoperative pain as well as the time required for hospitalization and related costs are reduced.

• In standard procedures, it is necessary to break the sternum and open the chest, which in turn causes severe pain in the shoulders and back, while in this method, only the wound related to the slit / 5. Up to 1 cm and a hole of 1 to 2 mm in the patient's back, which heals quickly.

• Skilled surgeons with unique capabilities will be available at more locations.

Disadvantages of Robotic method

• The greater the distance between the doctor and the patient, the slower the connection with equipment and monitors. Depending on the circumstances, physicians may experience a 25-second delay on monitors. These signs may mean death or life for the patient. These delays occur when the distance between the doctor and the patient is more than 90 miles. Need to improve the delay time between when the surgeon sees the knife move and when he actually makes the incision. This time should be less than one-fifth of a second, otherwise there is a possibility of cutting the wrong place. Currently the maximum distance a robot can operate is about 300 km (wired) or 35 km.

• The main obstacle to remote surgery is that it is a new technology and not all patients like to undergo such an operation.

• Robots are very expensive.

• The doctor does not have an assistant.

• Another problem is the lack of sensory feedback. In surgery, we usually understand how much the thread has been pulled by pulling the thread from the pressure on the hand, but here there is no more feedback and we have to measure the amount of tissue deformation. In the picture, he gained this understanding. However, learning this requires practice and courage, and of course puts a lot of pressure on the surgeon. Doctors who perform remote surgery cannot see the environment or feel what is happening around the patient because what is available to the doctor is video images.

Examples of surgical robots

1- ZeusT is a master-slave system that uses three robotic arms, two for transfer and work with surgical instruments and the other is a sound or foot-controlled endoscope. New ZeusT models have 5 degrees of freedom. The endoscope technology is called AESOP (Automated Endoscope System for Optimal Positioning). AESOP not only helps maintain a stable image of the surgical site but also eliminates the need for surgeon assistance. AESOP is very flexible with 6 degrees of freedom. The surgeon controls the ZeusT using the joysticks in each hand and looking at the TV screen. Joysticks are form-fitted to ensure that the surgeon's hand movements are correctly interpreted by ZeusT. The surgeon can see the image in 2 or 3 dimensions.

2- The da Vinci robot has three arms. One of the arms has a pair of miniature cameras that produce a three-dimensional image of the patient's body, which the surgeon sees on the monitor, and the other two arms, which perform surgery through small incisions just 8 mm wide.

The da Vinci surgical system is quite similar to the ZeusT model but does not have the AESOP voice recognition function. Da Vinci with 6 in freedom is more flexible than ZeusT. Da Vinci provides a three-dimensional image of the area.

3- Institute of Robotics and Mechatronics: The device made by this institute consists of a teleoperator and an operator console. The telecom operator consists of two Aesop robots (Computer Motion Inc.). One of the robots carries a surgical instrument equipped with a miniature force / torque sensor, and the other can perform a laparoscope. In the operator console, stereo video and measured power are both displayed. So the user not only sees, but also feels what is being done. A construction phantom (Sensible Technologies Inc) is used as a power display, and power information can be displayed visually if no tactile input is available.

UCB / UCSF laparoscopic telesurgical workstation

In this model, the slave manipulator is composed of two parts. The first part is responsible for determining the general location and is placed outside the body and is used to determine the position of the millibot. Millibot part II manipulators The first part has 4 in the direction of freedom. And since it is located outside the body, no hole has a size limit. The other end of this connection is a 4-piece connector. All 4 actuators involved in the overall positioning phase are DC servomotors. 2 is free and has a gripper on it. Its diameter is 15 mm and its length from Mag to Gripper is 5 cm. The master workstation consists of a pair of 6-degree free touch media that control each of the robotic arms. Phantom v1.5, Sensible Technologies Inc., Cambridge, MA) are designed to be kinematically similar to the structure of robotic arms.

Virtual Hospital

In the early 1990s, Finland faced the problem of the inability of the public health care system, on the other hand, to increase its aging population, prompting experts to find a way out of a possible crisis. In the fall of 1998, a small Finnish company decided to set up a medical counseling center and received treatment so that patients could communicate with skilled physicians around the world. The hospital network is only permanently accessible to those who have registered and paid a membership fee. After registration, patients will be able to benefit from medical advice. After registration, members are given an information card that identifies them as members of the orphanage. Due to security issues, the result of the consultation will not be sent by e-mail. And this is done over the phone. Members pay using the Scandinavian banking system or by credit card.

The services of this hospital are the possibility of accessing the drug database, internet chat and the possibility of receiving and storing information and adding information to the network. Patient information is protected by the SSL protocol, which is a secure way to transfer information, text, image, video and audio. The whole system also has very secret and protective layers that protect the network from the intrusion of others. There are concerns about using online clinical services, for example, patients may pretend to be ill to receive fake prescriptions. Therefore, it was decided not to prescribe strong drugs such as sleeping pills, sedatives or antibiotics based on online counseling. Research has shown that despite all the measures taken, half of the patients referred to the hospital were not really ill.

The first electronic hospital in Iran

The research project of the first electronic hospital in the country was put into operation on February 20, 2001 by the engineers of Arish Computer Software Company and under the supervision of Dr. Majdi, in Imam Hossein Teaching Hospital in Shahroud. This project was implemented at a cost of 880 million Rials over a period of 2 years and is now active around the clock in all departments of this hospital. Creating a fundamental change in hospital management and scientific management based on statistics and information, increasing speed and accuracy in providing services Improving the economics of treatment and providing quantitative and qualitative medical research is one of the goals of this project. The possibility of creating an electronic file for remote treatment of patients by internal and external physicians is another feature of this plan.

The hardware of this project includes 36 workstations with 2500 meters of cabling in a complex of 25,500 square meters of the hospital building and designing a speed of 100 MB per second and installing servers in the computer center and information center of the hospital. The software runs in a Windows environment and complies with international standards and is able to provide services in all departments of clinical, laboratory, radiology, operating rooms, emergency, office, medical records, pharmacies and warehouses.

This system has 46 computers, 11 printers of various types, video microscopes, digital cameras related to radiology scanners. The steps consist of 4 phases.

• Patient admission process until discharge.

• Paraclinics including pharmacy and pharmaceutical information, laboratories and wards, radiology and imaging.

• In sections including patient history, financial calculations, records. Pharmaceutical warehouses and...

• Management Support plan that includes management statistics, administrative affairs, consumer warehouses and property and workflow. And the last stage of the project is Telemedicine research and development.

The information of this system can be converted to Persian in other languages according to the information coding system

According to this plan and under a contract with the Ministry of Health, Treatment and Medical Education, in each of the provinces of the country, a hospital will be equipped with this system and the staff of the hospital will receive the necessary training. Currently, Vali-e-Asr (AS) hospitals in Zanjan and Baqiyatallah (AS) hospitals in Tehran are implementing this plan, and also in Imam Reza Hospital in Mashhad, the complete hospital network plan for the full implementation of this system is underway. In the provinces of West Azerbaijan and Yazd, the training of this project has been done.

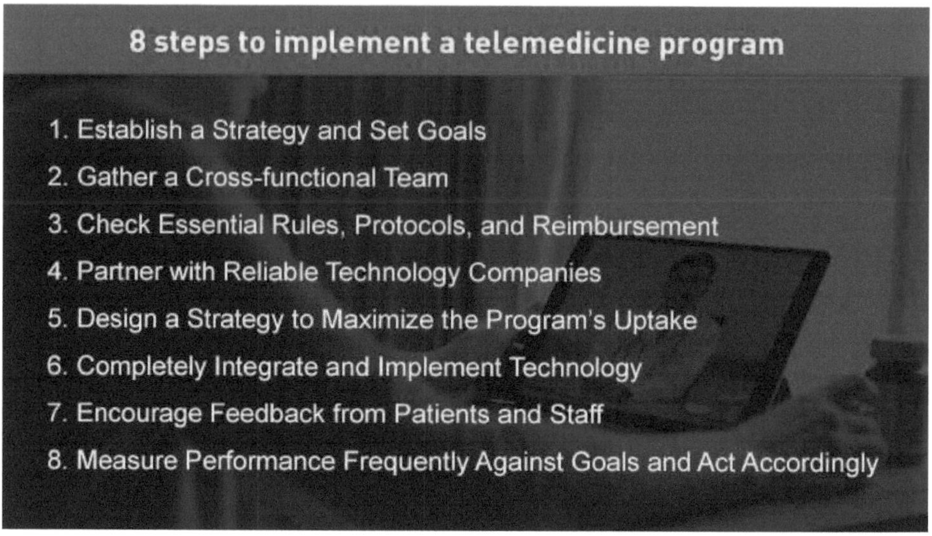

8 steps to implement a telemedicine program

1. Establish a Strategy and Set Goals
2. Gather a Cross-functional Team
3. Check Essential Rules, Protocols, and Reimbursement
4. Partner with Reliable Technology Companies
5. Design a Strategy to Maximize the Program's Uptake
6. Completely Integrate and Implement Technology
7. Encourage Feedback from Patients and Staff
8. Measure Performance Frequently Against Goals and Act Accordingly

Figure 41. Eight steps to implement a telemedicine program

It is expected that the hospitals equipped with this system will be connected to each other soon through the network of the Ministry of Health and it will be possible to exchange information throughout the country.

United Nations Telemedicine Project

The United Nations uses Telemedicine to monitor the situation of peacekeepers. Although soldiers undergo medical examinations and vaccinations before deployment, they are prone to indigenous diseases or accidents. Telecommunications infrastructure has been developed in the target areas, and as a result, soldiers can communicate with medical centers by telephone, fax, e-mail or teleconferencing. The scope of services includes medical consultation, medical and dental diagnoses, ECG, ENT and laboratory results, ultrasound and radiological images. Counseling will initially focus on cardiovascular disease and emergency patients, and then expand to the specialties of neurosurgery, orthopedics, skin diseases and other diseases.

Examples of equipment available at Telemedicine

The American TeleCare Telehealth system uses a regular telephone line to connect a Provider station to any number of patient video stations. A simple single-key activation provides communication between patients and the Health Center Provider with two-way, real-time communication capabilities via video monitor, camera, microphone and speaker. Two-way audio-visual communication with medical accessories provides a real-time picture of the patient's health status. Patient data is permanently stored in the Provider.

Other devices that this device can be equipped with:

• American TeleCare Care Tone Telephonic Stethoscope (standard).

• Blood Pressure and Pulse Meter (standard).

• Glucose Meter (optional).

• Pulse Oximeter (optional).

• Digital Scale (optional).

• PT / INR (optional).

• Digital Thermometer (optional).

Advantages of this system at a glance

• Ease of use.

• Ease of installation: Requires an analog telephone line and a grounded electrical outlet.

• Low volume and beautiful appearance.

Cybernet Medical Products

MedStar

It is a small and affordable device that collects, stores and sends vital data. Accessories are connected to color connectors and the whole unit is connected to a normal telephone line. The simple one-button function makes it easy for patients to use.

PAL Star

This allows hospital staff to ask patients remote questions. It is possible for patients to respond easily through contact pages. All information is transmitted through a regular telephone line. This device can be used alone or with MedStar.

Web System

MedStar and plaster devices are supported by a powerful, easy-to-use web-based medical database. Reports, alerts, and data analysis components are available in this environment.

Vitaphone made of element can record data related to heart activity and send it to the doctor when it is pressed to a patient's chest. For the first time in the world, the Vitaphone 2300 (Cardio Phone) provides the ability to record, store and transmit digital 3-channel ecg via mobile phone without the need for cables or adhesive electrodes. With the push of a button, the ecg registration is started and it happens completely automatically. Sending ecg to Vitaphone Medical Center is the same. A GPS receiver inside the Vitaphone 2300 also helps determine the exact position of the patient in an emergency.

LifeShirt is a wearable, mesh-like, lightweight blouse with sensors built into it for continuous collection and monitoring of more than 30 physiological indicators, including respiration and phlebic activity and other physiological parameters. Data is sent through handsets for monitoring by medical personnel.

4- Scientists at the University of Bristol have built a Cyberjacket, which is actually a wearable computer system. It has three sensors: a temperature sensor, an ECG and an oxygen saturation monitor. It is also equipped with GPS to determine the position and uses the accelerometer for motion sensation. The Cyberjacket architecture is modular in design. Researchers can easily customize and customize a jacket for their own experiments.

This cover system has a processor unit and a 9-wire bus that is embedded in the fabric of the jacket. This bus provides the energy required by the sensors and their ground and connections and communications through three serial links. Two of the links in the levels RS-232 runs and is dedicated to RS-232 devices. Any commercial inventory that implements rs-232s (such as GPS) can be connected to one of these buses. The third bass is implemented at the TTL level with a volume of 4800 and various devices such as medical sensors can be connected to it. In addition, bitsy can produce stereo audio feedback that can be used to give feedback to the person wearing the clothes. If the doctor wants to contact the patient remotely, he can do so through a microphone-speaker installed inside the garment. The patient's position can be found quickly and accurately by GPS, if necessary. This dress should be comfortable and ergonomic.

Concluding remarks

In the last decade, many advances have been made in the development of telemedicine technology as a method of telemedicine care supported by modern digital media communications. In many countries, the medical care system is getting closer to the patient. Especially telemedicine in countries such as Iran, where the transportation network is less developed, the dispersion of the population in some parts of the country and mountainous and impassable areas, lack of access to specialized medical centers in many parts of the country and the aging population and Requires intensive medical care, greatly helps in the rapid diagnosis of the disease, adopts the correct treatment tactics, reduces waste of time (which in some cases is vital, such as heart disease) and reduces the associated costs (direct and indirect). The relentless growth of technology and public access to communication and computer systems have opened new horizons in medical science and made the impossible possible.

1- In today's world, despite significant advances in medicine, heart disease is still an important issue and a common cause of death for patients. In our country, according to statistics published by Behesht Zahra, 18674 residents of Tehran died of heart attack in 1996. According to doctors, ECG is still the most useful way to diagnose heart disease. Due to the importance of this issue, in today's advanced societies, increasing attention is paid to electrocardiographic systems. The task of these systems is to receive the patient's heart signals and send them through communication lines to a hospital or specialized clinic. This reduces waste of time and quickly assesses the patient's condition. In this case, the patient is able to communicate with a specialist in different physical and mental situations. In Iran, the design and construction of a telephone system for sending heart signals has been done successfully. The system designer (Jalil Mazlum) suggests upgrading the system to the ability to send other important clinical parameters such as blood pressure, heart rate and respiratory volume.

Advances in communication technology and medical care programs and monitoring devices of vital factors promise us to increase the quality of medical care at home. With the establishment of a remote counseling system and the availability of vital factor monitoring devices in the patient, hospital, specialized clinic or family doctor can always take care of their patients and in any case provide the necessary advice and instructions. And if necessary, issue an order for rapid transfer of the patient to an equipped medical center. Medical centers, being aware of the patient's condition, can prepare the patient for admission in order to implement the treatment as soon as possible. Patient monitoring in their homes is considered to be one of the largest markets in the next decade.

The connection between specialized hospitals in big cities for consulting in different fields of medicine and management will be a great help in improving the patient's treatment, reducing costs and traffic load. This relationship speeds up the diagnosis and treatment more accurately by exchanging views and collaborating with relevant medical professionals in hospitals. Hospitals can also find out about each other's conditions, such as the availability of medical specialties needed for emergencies or the number of vacant beds at any one time.

The existence of a communication line between the hospital and the specialist, the information about the patient's condition in case of emergency can be sent to the doctor at home or at work immediately. Depending on the equipment available, this information could be ECG, radiographs, or ultrasound. In this case, the doctor can provide the necessary recommendations and, if necessary, take you to the hospital.

Due to the lack of some specialties or the high cost of treatment in many northern neighboring countries, with the establishment of a medical communication channel, the field of cooperation, exchange of views and, if necessary, transfer of patients to specialized hospitals in Iran can be directed. This issue is especially useful for patients in need of open-heart surgery and due to the existence of highly experienced cardiac surgery specialists in Iran, in terms of income.

During the tourism season, the number of people living in tourist islands increases sharply. In order to respond to the demand for specialized medical services in emergency and daily cases, it is necessary to establish a permanent connection between the medical centers of these points and the main hospitals in the motherland and reduce the risk and costs of transferring the patient to the mainland. This plan also suggests the possibility of communicating with medical centers in other countries. This is especially important for foreigners during the tourism season. Because they can communicate with medical professionals who speak their own language. In addition, local medical officials can obtain the patient's clinical history from the patient's country of origin. (In this regard, establishing a telemedicine network in important tourist cities of Iran such as Isfahan, Shiraz and Yazd, for the comfort and safety of more tourists in terms of attracting tourists, will not be useless.) Significant reduction of time for diagnosis is a great advantage It is especially valuable for patients with myocardial infarction. In this case, the implementation of the rapid germination method significantly increases the patient's chances of survival.

Establishing a system of telemedicine counseling at sea is recommended due to Iran's abundant maritime relations with neighboring countries and the existence of passenger ships in the Caspian Sea, using satellite communications. Also, a system similar to the above method can be used for medical advice on the plane in case of emergency.

Establishing a telemedicine network in large areas with low population density (such as the eastern and southeastern regions of the country) as well as in mountainous and impassable areas due to the very poor development of the transportation network, especially during emergencies.

Establishing a telemedicine network in relation to veterans and the disabled in relation to the transportation problems of these people seems to be very useful. In this case, the relevant medical centers or doctors can take care of them on a regular basis and, if necessary, provide the necessary advice and counseling.

The implementation of automated health laboratory systems in the country is a big step towards achieving public welfare, so that by covering the majority of the community, especially villagers, and reducing costs and saving time, it has ensured and controlled the health of the statistical community. In addition, it improves the quality of e-government services and increases the country's competitiveness and increases the level of use among countries in the region. ICT provides facilities for creating e-health geographic maps using data obtained from the intelligent system of the automated laboratory system for e-government to directly examine and record the quantity and quality of various blood factors in different parts of the country. Create medical dynamic records, retrieve maps continuously. This allows a specific area to be identified in terms of blood health and its drug and medical needs to be identified and the effects of the measures taken to be examined with each test plan.

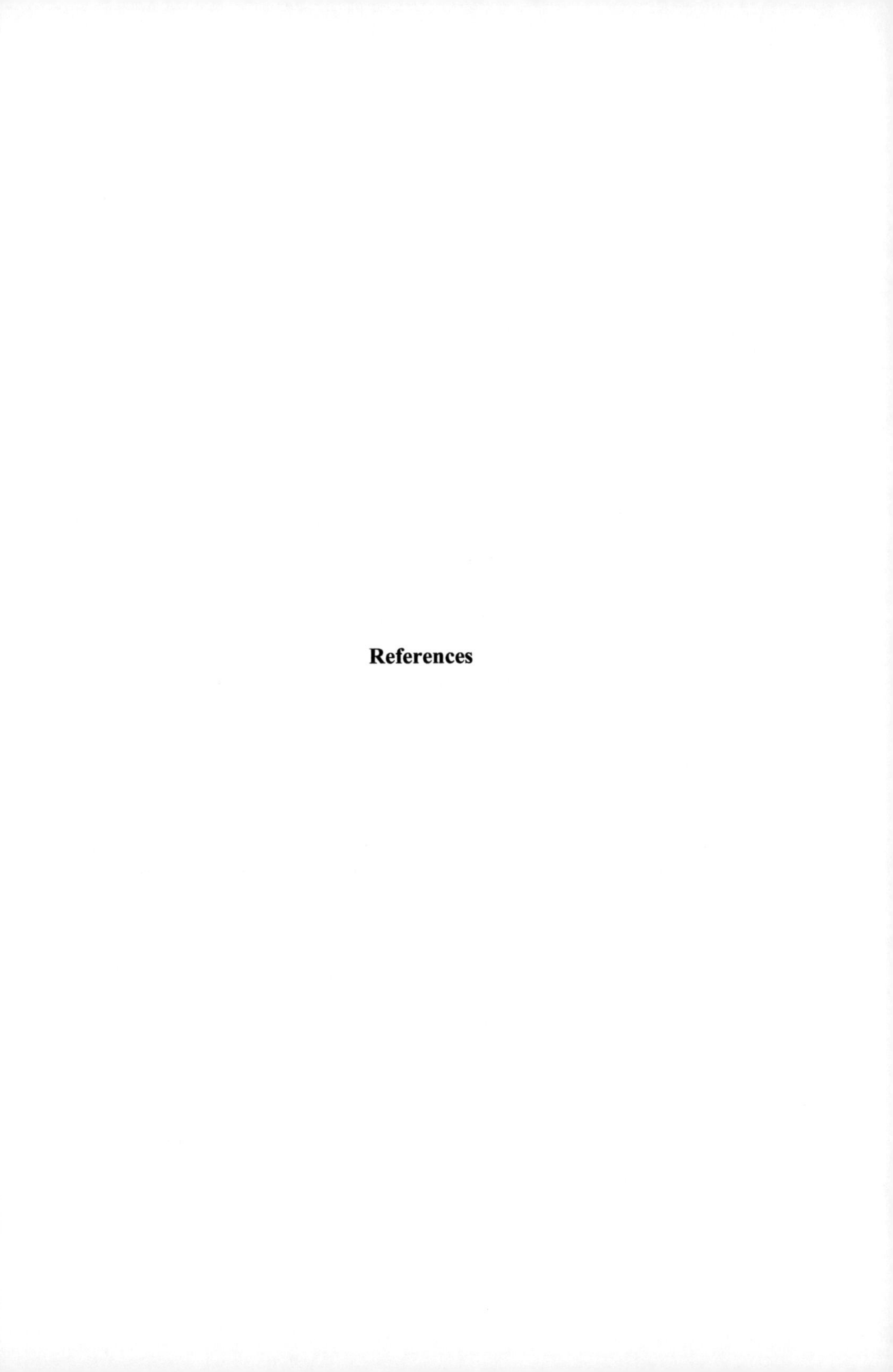

References

Eu.bac product certification “Building automation impact on energy efficiency,” Application per EN 15232.

Chen-xu Liu, Qing-An Zeng, Yun Liu, “A Dynamic Load Control Scheme Grid Systems,” ElSEVIER, pp. 200–205, Sep. 30, 2011.

Principles and foundations of intelligent control systems and BMS, authored by Rasoul Haddadi Nistanak

Organization Theory (Structure, Design, Applications) Stephen Robbins - Translated by Dr. Seyed Mehdi Alvani and Hassan Danaeifard - Second Edition 1999 - Safar Publications

Instructions for submitting medical records and information, Ministry of Health and Medical Education, Deputy of Treatment, Office of Hospital Management and Clinical Services Excellence, Code of National Instruction A-P-7-3-35-1695

Dr. Mousavi. SA, Frvghy.syd, Zekavati. Roya, Mousavi. Fatemeh, Principles and Principles of Management in Nursing, Publisher of Ashura Institute 2014

Dogas.Borley Witter. Principles of patient care..Volume one. Translated by Forouzan Atashzadeh. Shorideh and ... Golban. Tehran 2012

Shidfar, Mohammad Reza. Comprehensive book of public health. Volume one, second edition of the Ministry of Health, Medical Education / Deputy of Research and Technology.2010

Salavati, Mojgan, Yazdandoost, Rangar, (2010). Schema therapy, faculty publication, first edition.

Salavati, M. (2007). Dominant Schemas and the Effectiveness of Schema Therapy in Female Patients with Borderline Personality Disorder, PhD Thesis in Clinical Psychology, Tehran Institute of Psychiatry, Iran School of Medical Sciences.

Azimi, Sirus; Principles of General Psychology, Tehran, Saffar, 2014, 16th edition, pp. 24, 25, 26.

Farhadian, Reza. (376 1). Personality Theory, Binat, Vol. 14, pp. 15-20 ...

Carol, Taylor, Principles of Nursing Taylor: Nursing Concepts, translated by Zahra Safavi Bayat, The Honorary Legend of Manesh and Others. Human Publishing, Second Edition, 2010.

Kaplan, Herlod, Zadok, Benjamin. (2010). Summary of Psychiatric Behavioral Sciences - Clinical Psychiatry, Volume I, Tabriz Shahrab Water Publishing.

Karimi, Yousef (2001). "Personality Psychology", Nazar Editing Institute, p. 5

Keith, m. David Sun. (2004). Application of cognitive therapy in personality disorders (translated by Shams, Giti). Tehran: Roshd Publications

Human Resource Management - Dr. Esfandiar Saadat - Samat Publications - Fourth Edition 2000

Human Resource Management in Employee Affairs - Dr. Seyed Javadin - Second Edition - Negah Dash Publications 2003

Masoudi Asl. Yerevan, Principles of Nursing Services Management, Second Edition, Jame Negar Publisher, 2016

Mossadegh Rad, Ali Mohammad. (2003). The role of participatory management (suggestion system) in the effectiveness and efficiency of the hospital, Journal of Research in Medical Sciences, Isfahan University of Medical Sciences, 8 (3): 89-85.

Mossadegh Rad, Ali Mohammad. (2004). Investigating the Relationship between Employees' Job Satisfaction with the Management Style of Managers of University Hospitals in Isfahan, Journal of Humanities and Social Sciences, Mazandaran University, 4 (12): 143-169.

Mossadegh Rad, Ali Mohammad. Textbook of Hospital Organization and Specialized Management (2), Dibagaran Publications, Tehran, 2004

Mossadegh Rad, Ali Mohammad. Generalities of Health Organization and Management, Dibagaran Publications, Tehran, 2015

Mossadegh Rad, Ali Mohammad. Generalities of Health Services Management, Dibagaran Publications, Tehran, 2002

Hrvabady.shfyqh, Morbagh. Akram, Nursing and Midwifery Management, Publisher of Iranian Medical Sciences and Health Services, Second Edition, 2006

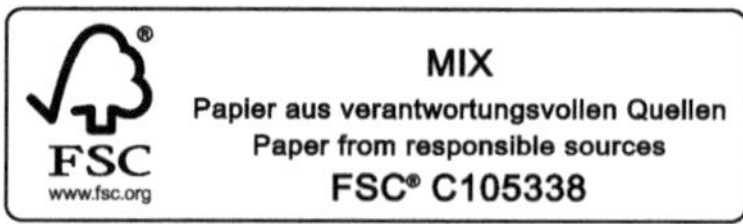

Printed by Books on Demand GmbH, Norderstedt / Germany